T0190766

YOUR

BRAIN

ON

PREGNANCY

A Guide to Understanding and Protecting Your
Mental Health During Pregnancy and Beyond

Dr. Dawn Kingston, PhD

Published by Simon & Schuster

NEW YORK • LONDON • TORONTO
SYDNEY • NEW DELHI

SIMON &
SCHUSTER
CANADA

A Division of Simon & Schuster, LLC
166 King Street East, Suite 300
Toronto, Ontario M5A 1J3

This Simon & Schuster Canada edition September 2024

SIMON & SCHUSTER CANADA and colophon are trademarks of Simon & Schuster, LLC

Simon & Schuster: Celebrating 100 Years of Publishing in 2024

For information about special discounts for bulk purchases, please contact Simon & Schuster Special Sales at 1-800-268-3216 or CustomerService@simonandschuster.ca.

Manufactured in the United States of America

1   3   5   7   9   10   8   6   4   2

Library and Archives Canada Cataloguing in Publication
Title: Your brain on pregnancy : a guide to understanding and protecting your mental health during pregnancy and beyond / Dawn Kingston.
Names: Kingston, Dawn, author.
Description: Simon & Schuster Canada edition.
Identifiers: Canadiana (print) 20210241659 | Canadiana (ebook) 20210241853 |
ISBN 9781982143374 (softcover) | ISBN 9781982143381 (ebook)
Subjects: LCSH: Pregnancy—Psychological aspects—Popular works. | LCSH: Childbirth—Psychological aspects—Popular works. | LCSH: Motherhood—Psychological aspects—Popular works. | LCSH: Pregnant women—Mental health—Popular works. | LCSH: Mothers—Mental health—Popular works.
Classification: LCC RG560 .K56 2022 | DDC 618.2001/9—dc23

ISBN 978-1-9821-4337-4
ISBN 978-1-9821-4338-1 (ebook)

I dedicate this book to my husband, Robert, and my sons, Joshua and Joel, who have blessed me with unspeakable joy

Contents

YOUR
BRAIN
ON
PREGNANCY

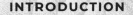

First Steps

"Congratulations! You must be so happy! You're absolutely glowing."

How many times have we heard these words being said to a woman who is pregnant? Or maybe we've said them ourselves? Family, friends, colleagues, social media, television, and certainly most pregnancy books all tell us that pregnant women are radiant, healthy, and happy. When I was pregnant with our first son, I was full of anticipation. Our second pregnancy was the same. *What will this new baby be like?* I wondered. *How will our lives be different?* There were the usual worries, but overall, I had a sense of hope and promise about our future as a new family.

Pregnancy can be a time of excitement, possibility, and growth. The future is full of bright plans. Perhaps you've been dreaming about this moment for years. Perhaps you've struggled to conceive, and you're overjoyed to finally be pregnant. Perhaps this is an opportunity to bring you and your partner closer together, to grow your family.

Of course, there are times when not everything is rosy. I've been there, and I'm sure you have, too. Perhaps you've had a concern that you can't seem to shake, or you've been more irritable and edgier than usual. Maybe you've been feeling down and out of sorts. Many pregnant women experience temporary mood swings or teariness that come upon them out of the blue—often at the most inconvenient times! These are a normal part of pregnancy, and while some women experience them more often and intensely than others, they pass after a few minutes or hours. But for some women, pregnancy is a time of *constant* worry, stress, and even sadness.

I've been working with women and babies for over thirty years, as a registered nurse in neonatal intensive care units, a mental health clinician, and a researcher specializing in women's mental health, and what I've discovered is that mental health challenges *during* pregnancy (prenatal) are much more common than we think. The findings from my team of researchers at the University of Calgary—and other researchers around the world—tell the unspoken and dramatic story that as many as 1 in 4 pregnant women struggle with their emotional health worldwide.[1, 2, 3] What stands out to me is that this statistic is universal. When we conduct research, we often see different rates of illnesses and diseases depending on the country. But the rate of prenatal mental health problems is consistent across the globe, showing us both that they are commonly experienced by women across the world *and* what causes them is common.

I have always been passionate about serving mothers and babies. My journey as a researcher in this field began when I was a neonatal nurse caring for sick and preterm infants in neonatal ICUs and tertiary care centers at hospitals across Ontario, including St. Joseph's Hospital in London and McMaster University Medical Center in Hamilton. I had a special interest in supporting families who were facing loss or challenges, such as new, uncertain diagnoses or poor prognosis of sick or preterm babies, and as a result, I was often given assignments where I helped families through challenging, often tragic, situations. But as valuable and impactful as this help was, I couldn't help but wonder how we could prevent these events in the first place.

These experiences solidified my desire to improve the lives of mothers and their babies, and at the time there was a lot of focus and research on the toxic effects of stress around pregnancy, birth, and postpartum. After my master's in nursing, where I focused on helping new mothers build confidence around breastfeeding, I went on to do my PhD in nursing and decided to study the predictors of stress in pregnancy and the link between stress and preterm birth. There was a growing group of researchers and clinicians who were interested in how to prevent preterm birth. I wanted to be a part of the worldwide effort to answer the question, How do we lower the risk of a mother delivering a baby early?

That was the starting point of my doctoral dissertation. I immediately came toe-to-toe with three decades of research of animal and human studies that link stress to preterm birth, but what I quickly discovered was that it wasn't just *stress* that was implicated in preterm birth—it was the breadth of prenatal mental health problems that impacted the baby's well-being. And preterm birth wasn't the only outcome of prenatal mental health problems—there were a host of other long-term developmental, physical, neurodevelopmental, and mental health outcomes, such as obesity, diabetes, heart disease, autism, attention deficit/hyperactivity disorder, childhood anxiety and depression, and sleep and behavioural difficulties.

I've always been a big-system, visionary thinker. As I looked at our North American health care systems, I was dismayed that there wasn't routine screening or mental health care offered to women during their thirteen visits of prenatal care. After all, pregnancy was a time when women would experience regular, intensive contact with the medical system. In my mind, the mismatch between the clear evidence that prenatal mental health problems contribute to significant, long-standing developmental, physical, and mental health challenges in children and the lack of a response by the system (implementing preventive and ameliorative health care) was inexcusable, especially given the awareness about postpartum depression (depression after pregnancy, also known as PPD). We hear about PPD all the time—in books, on television, in the news, in prenatal classes, and from our doctors and nurses—but we rarely hear about the mental health problems that can occur *during pregnancy* that have a dual effect on mother-to-be and baby, like depression, anxiety, and stress.

Women see health care providers during pregnancy more regularly than almost any other time in their lives. During prenatal visits, women undergo physical exams, ultrasounds, and laboratory tests that screen for physical conditions such as diabetes, high blood pressure, infection, and fetal anomalies, but these are far less common than mental health problems. Yet rarely are a few minutes devoted to asking simple screening questions that would identify the most common mental health problems in pregnancy. Our health care system wasn't serving mothers, so I set out to find how to fix it.

In 2011, I traveled to Australia as a postdoctoral fellow to meet with clinicians, researchers, policymakers, and decision makers to understand how Australia managed to design and implement a national perinatal mental health program. (When it comes to mental health and pregnancy, we use the term *perinatal mental health*, with *perinatal* referring to the period of time between when you become pregnant and up to a year after giving birth.) When I came back to Canada, I began working with the Lois Hole Hospital for Women in Edmonton to conduct research into the systemic barriers that deterred (1) health care workers in Canada from providing mental health screening and referral care and (2) women from sharing their mental health concerns with their doctors. We conducted hundreds of surveys, asking women what their experience was with mental health and in the health care system, working with physicians, midwives, and others. And what we found was that we were in a catch-22 cycle.

My research team has coined the phrase, "Women don't tell, and providers don't ask." Over 75 percent of pregnant women in our studies told us that the biggest barrier to talking about mental health was not knowing what is "normal" and "not normal" during pregnancy. One of the myths about pregnancy is that all emotional vulnerability is due to hormone fluctuations, and is normal, random, and uncontrollable. One of the aims of this book is to disrupt that myth so that you understand exactly what causes mental health suffering and what you can do about it.

Sometimes there are deep, unspoken reasons that keep women from reaching out, such as feeling ashamed for having a mental health problem or guilty for failing to meet the expectations of what a mother-to-be should be feeling—happy and rosy. As a result, many women suffer in silence, wrestling with deep sadness and unrelenting worry and wondering: *What's wrong with me? Am I crazy? Am I not a good mom? Am I damaging my child? Will I ruin my child and her future?* Unacknowledged, these feelings snowball, creating a cycle of guilt, confusion—and powerlessness and hopelessness. And if a woman doesn't realize that she is suffering, it's unlikely that anyone else—including her partner or her doctor—will detect her symptoms and even unlikelier that she will reach out for help herself.[4]

The statistics here are dire: only 30 percent to 50 percent of pregnant women with depression, anxiety, or stress are identified as having symptoms, and fewer than 20 percent receive mental health care.[5] The evidence worldwide points to insufficient resources to help people to manage and recover from mental health problems. Indeed, not one country has ever reached the point of having enough mental health resources, and decision makers remain stuck at the planning stage without good solutions to offer.[6]

A major part of our research and others' has been to understand what holds women back from getting help for depression, anxiety, and stress so that we can help to make the journey easier.[7, 8, 9, 10] In addition to not knowing what is normal and not normal, 70 percent of women are hesitant to talk to their prenatal provider about their mental health concerns because they wanted to handle their mental health concerns on their own or with their partner/friend/family member. Forty-four percent were worried about being put on antidepressants, and 46 percent believed that their symptoms would get better on their own. I include these percentages because I want you to see just how many women feel this way.

On the other side, we found that 98 percent of women were happy to disclose their mental health concerns when they knew help was available and their prenatal provider was interested, sensitive, and caring. Ninety-five percent were reassured when told there were many options for help—not just medication—and 88 percent when they heard other woman also struggled in a similar way.[11]

The findings of our research and the results from the Australian trip meant only one thing: It would take years to fix the medical system—and we didn't have that kind of time.

We needed to put women in the driver's seat of their own mental health care.

Through my work with the University of Alberta, the Lois Hole Hospital for Women, and the University of Calgary, where I am a provincial research chair in women's mental health, my team and I have created a platform called Hope, a digital platform that provides women with free resources to manage their own mental health. In other words, giving women in Canada the same opportunities they get elsewhere to bypass the system and manage their own mental health. We conducted research using the UK's ALSPAC study (Avon Longitudinal Study of Parents and Children), the largest database of research about women and mothers that has been following women through pregnancy and their kids since the early 1990s. We don't have the same longitudinal research in Canada, though Australia and several Nordic countries also do it. Needless to say, this research that allows us to understand challenges in women's and children's lives is an invaluable resource.

Over the past decade, awareness has started to grow, and there's a burgeoning concern about the number of pregnant women struggling with their mental health. Mental health problems are now recognized as one of the top three complications of pregnancy because we've found that, without treatment, these problems can continue for years, affecting the mother's long-term mental health as well as her baby's mental health and development.

As parents, we want to set our children up for success, but these complications can make it difficult for us to parent the way we want to. They can cause our relationships with our partner, friends, and family to suffer, limiting the very supports that could help us. Mental health problems are like a pebble dropped into a pond, and the ripples that stone creates are like the wide-reaching effects of letting these issues go untreated.

But it doesn't have to be that way. New neuroscientific research has created a seismic shift in the way we view and treat mental health problems, opening the door for us to interrupt the cycle of prenatal mental health problems.

We know now that mental health problems result when our brain and nervous system become dysregulated, most often by difficult life circumstances that we faced—in childhood or adulthood. In other words, symptoms of depression, anxiety, and stress are not life sentences. They are like a fever—a sign of a dysregulated brain and nervous system. They signal to us that we've experienced a significant event, and our body has taken a hit. In this book, I lay out the evidence of how overwhelming situations jar our nervous system into dysregulation—and how simple, highly effective tools can re-regulate your nervous system and reduce your mental health symptoms.

The first step is getting rid of that shame, guilt, and embarrassment. Underlying many of the reasons that hold women back from getting help is the stigma that while it is perfectly acceptable to be diagnosed with a physical ailment like diabetes, it is only the broken, weak, inferior, defective, and incompetent who suffer with a mental health problem. But that's not the case with dysregulation, which is a physical ailment with a physical solution, just like diabetes.

As we enter into this new, neuroscience-based paradigm in perinatal mental health, I hope that the intractable problem of access to care will shift, that we will see healthier mothers and healthier babies, taking the pressure off our neonatal intensive care units and children's mental health services. I hope that we will no longer need to ask the question, "What holds you back from getting mental health care?" because women will have the tools at their fingertips.

In the spirit of empowering women to care for their own mental health, I wrote this book.

We'll start with the research into main causes and risk factors for mental health problems in pregnancy, the evidence about the consequences for mother and baby, and the exciting and hopeful new research about strategies that can reverse these consequences. I'll walk you through the foundations of mental health, then I'll discuss what depression, anxiety, and toxic stress in pregnancy look like, describe what warning signs and symptoms to be mindful of, share tools that you can use to do a personal self-assessment of where you are at, and give you practical techniques for improving your mental health. I'll also provide you with the most recent evidence on advantages and disadvantages of taking antidepressants before, during, and after pregnancy. You don't have to read this book from start to finish. I invite you to dip in and out of the chapters as you need.

Throughout the book, I've included vignettes that are inspired by real women who I've encountered in my research and clinical practice. These stories are not unique, because the struggles are not unique. They are shared by women the world over, but I include them here because there is comfort in knowing that others share our pain and struggles and to show you that there is hope. These are women just like you who have navigated the journey of mental health suffering and stepped onto a path of wellness and thriving.

A note on terminology: In this book, I use the term *women* to refer to all people who identify as women, but this book is also for pregnant partners for whom this book's content on pregnancy is found helpful.

My wish for you is that the strategies outlined here will help you alleviate any distress you may currently be experiencing and manage your mental health so you can enjoy your pregnancy and move forward in this new stage of your life with energy, optimism, joy, and confidence. But I also hope that these techniques will become part of the fabric of your life beyond your pregnancy and help you, your partner, and your children continue your journey of emotional and mental health and resiliency in the years to come.

CHAPTER 1

The Research

For a long time, we in the medical profession viewed depression in the postnatal period, or postpartum depression, as the main perinatal mental health problem. But the accumulation of research over the past decade tells us that mental health problems in the prenatal period (during pregnancy) are just as common, and it isn't just depression—anxiety and toxic stress are real and growing challenges.

As I mentioned in the introduction, 1 in 4 pregnant women struggle with their mental health, with the primary issues being depression, anxiety, and toxic stress. Drilling down, studies show that 10 percent to 25 percent of women experience symptoms of prenatal depression. An intriguing report from the Avon Longitudinal Study of Parents and Children cohort, a landmark study that has collected data on pregnant women and their children since the early 1990s, showed an increase in rates of prenatal depression since the study's inception. For example, 17 percent of women had prenatal depression in 1991–92, and 25 percent of *their* daughters experienced symptoms when assessed in 2018. The investigators concluded that prenatal depression is 51 percent more common now than it was twenty-five years ago, which is consistent with trends of increasing mental health problems across the globe.[1] For prenatal anxiety, recent compilations of research report rates of 20 percent to 21 percent, with rates of stress high enough to be linked to adverse infant outcomes at well over 50 percent.[2]

In this chapter, I'll discuss what causes these mental health problems in pregnancy, what risk factors to be mindful of, and the pushback factors that can help alleviate symptoms. I'll also describe the consequences of depression, anxiety, and stress for mother and baby so that you are empowered to take steps to better your mental health.

Causes of Mental Health Problems in Pregnancy

It is our deeply human curiosity and creativity that leads us to wonder what the cause of illness is. All health issues, including mental health problems, have two parts: causes and risk factors. *Causes* are the fundamental underlying processes that start the process of illness moving and that ultimately lead to the manifestation of symptoms of disease. *Risk factors* are the things that create the fertile milieu for the underlying cause to take hold and grow. It's important to know the difference between them because, while you don't always have control over the causes of illness, you can absolutely manage your risk factors.

Let me use an example of the flu. The flu is *caused* by a virus. Without the virus, you would not develop the flu. But just having the virus doesn't mean you'll develop flu symptoms. You may be in optimal physical health so that your body mounts an immune response and eliminates the virus without you knowing you had it.

However, being physically depleted and under stress are *risk factors* that make you more vulnerable to getting the flu because your body is less capable of fighting it. They influence whether the virus in your body becomes a full-blown flu or something that your body handles quietly without you even being aware of it.

Many people think that prenatal and postpartum depression are caused by hormonal changes that women experience in pregnancy and post-birth, but pregnancy hormones play a very small part. In truth, the exact causes aren't known, but as with the vast majority of health challenges most researchers and clinicians recognize, there isn't one single explanation. Years of research have brought us to the consensus that prenatal mental health problems emerge when a *biological vulnerability* (or biological cause) is triggered by difficult life circumstances. In other words, we possess a susceptibility to a mental health problem that, like the flu virus, may or may not ever result in us developing depression or anxiety in our lives.

And we are not always born with biological vulnerabilities. Some develop during our lifetime, usually at the hands of challenging life circumstances. This principle, that "An individual's experience can shape their own neurobiology over time," is well accepted now, founded on three decades of stress and neuroscience research.[3] We're starting to see this principle emerge in the clinical world, too, although there is room to improve the practical application. For example, it would be ideal if each time we sought help from our medical professional for a physical issue, our visit included mental health screening.

The three main vulnerabilities that have the strongest impact on our mental health are a dysregulated nervous system, genetics, and personality traits. When these three vulnerabilities are present, adverse life experiences have the potential to increase our risk of mental health problems.

Dysregulated Nervous System

Let's start with a few basics: our nervous system includes the brain, spinal cord, and the complex network of nerves that send messages back and forth between the brain and the body and is the study of neuroscience. Thanks to an explosion of neuroscientific research in the last decades, our thinking about good mental health has shifted. We now know that one of the foundations of good mental health is a regulated nervous system, which means mental health problems arise when that system becomes dysregulated.

Regulation versus Dysregulation

Safety is the language of our nervous system. The brain and nervous system are regulated when they sense safety and dysregulated when they detect inescapable danger. Picture a lighthouse set high upon a rocky cliff, its large, bright light rotating around all night long so that ships can detect and avoid danger. Our brain does the same thing: it is constantly scanning our environment for things that could harm us, and it is doing so in a stealth manner, far below the surface of conscious awareness.

When it does detect a threat, our brain protects us by sending a signal to our body to respond to danger in a way that will keep us safe and intact. This is called a stress response: our muscles tense, our heart rate increases, our breathing quickens, and our pupils dilate, all to prepare us to physically move to a place of safety. Our nervous system is in good working order when it reacts to an immediate threat for a period of seconds or minutes and then calms down again, having done its job to protect us and remove us from danger.

However, when we live in a continuous state of threat and danger (e.g., being in an abusive relationship, working in a toxic work culture), our nervous system doesn't have the opportunity to de-escalate. It's always on, constantly detecting and warning us of imminent danger, and we don't experience the normal recovery period that our brain, nervous system, and body require. It's dysregulated—no longer operating in the optimal range.

Simply put, our brain and nervous system are designed to react and recover. When confronted with danger, our brain and nervous system mobilize body systems to enable us to escape the danger. Danger behind us, our brain, nervous system, and body then recover and return to normal parameters. When we are dysregulated, we react—but we don't recover. This dysregulation manifests as:

- feeling agitated or on edge, worried, panicked, anxious, and/or stressed
- feeling emotionally fragile, confused, or off-balance
- feeling frustrated or angry
- experiencing distress in relationships
- having greater vulnerability to illness (getting sick more often, high blood pressure, heart disease, weight gain, headache, memory impairment, shoulder and back tension, stomach and digestive problems)
- being distracted, unable to focus, having difficulty concentrating and an inability to follow through
- feeling depressed
- having low energy, needing to conserve energy
- poor sleeping (having trouble getting to, or staying, asleep)
- feeling the world is dangerous, chaotic, and unfriendly[4, 5]

Our nervous system can become dysregulated when we face any kind of an event or circumstance in our lives—in childhood or adulthood—that leads us to feel unsafe, threatened, in danger, powerless (as if we cannot escape), and overwhelmed (because it seems beyond our ability to manage the situation). A recent review paper listed more than fifty life circumstances that have the potential to dysregulate our nervous system, including the onset of a new illness, death of a significant other, loss of a parent, abortion/miscarriage, social isolation, migration, an education setback, a major change in living conditions, work loss, shift work, and retirement, to name but a few.[6] Dysregulation can also result from a significant one-time event, like a car accident, or a long-lasting circumstance, such as living in an abusive household or being raised by an alcoholic parent.

What causes a difficult life situation to turn into a dysregulating, neurobiologically jarring event is when it bears the features of feeling dangerous and inescapable. We might not *be* in actual danger, but we *feel* all the symptoms as if we were. At this point, the experience literally becomes embedded in our nervous system, shifting the wiring of our brain circuits and nervous system.[7] This rewiring primes our nervous system to be alerted to respond to any sort of triggers that mimic that original situation that created the initial impact. For instance, if you were in a car accident, you might find yourself feeling anxious with gut tensing and heart racing any time that you drove past the accident site—or any other location that even looked remotely similar to the site, had the same lighting conditions, smelled or sounded the same. Your brain is doing exactly what it should be doing—alerting you to danger at the site and giving you all the signals to *get away now*. When your nervous system is dysregulated, it can't distinguish between the "that was then" and "this is now."

Nervous system dysregulation shows up on all levels—emotionally (what we feel), physically (what we experience in our bodies), behaviourally (what we do), cognitively (what we think), relationally (how we show up in relationships), and what we believe and think about the world around us (we distrust, don't expect others to protect us, believe it is our fault, expect bad things to continue, etc.).[8]

Clinical psychologist Dr. Janina Fisher calls signs of dysregulation "the living legacy of trauma," and has identified eighteen physical and emotional symptoms that arise after the experience of a traumatic event. Many people don't recognize that these symptoms are a "legacy" or "carryover" of their experience, so in her work as a trauma expert, Dr. Fisher asks her clients to identify all of the symptoms they experience so they can understand how these responses helped them cope with the aftermath of their experience at one time but are no longer beneficial in their lives now.

If you are suffering from the aftermath of a difficult event or circumstance, take this opportunity to note all the symptoms that you experience:

depression
irritability
decreased concentration
numbing
loss of interest, defeat, resignation
insomnia
emotional overwhelm
loss of a sense of the future, hopelessness
shame and worthlessness
few or no memories
nightmares, flashbacks
hypervigilance, mistrust
anxiety, panic attacks
chronic pain, headaches
substance abuse, eating disorders

feeing unreal or out of body

self-destructive behaviour

loss of sense of "who I am"[9]

The more symptoms that you identified with, the more likely your life has been impacted by a past experience and the greater the chance that your brain and nervous system are dysregulated. If you circled several symptoms and you find it difficult to just get through the day most days in a week, consider reaching out to a therapist who specializes in trauma.

Our nervous system can be jarred into long-term dysregulation by overwhelming adversity that happens to us *at any point of our lives*—as infants in the womb, children, adolescents, or adults—and it can involve a one-time event or an ongoing situation. This is why having skills to re-regulate our nervous system is critical. However, we are most prone to dysregulation when we experience hardship during the critical or sensitive periods of our lives when our brain and nervous system are growing rapidly and are therefore particularly sensitive to injury and disruption, such as in utero, childhood (especially the first five years), and adolescence.[10]

Fetal development is the first critical period of our lives. For the past three decades, a large body of international research has proven that the prenatal environment affects our risk for lifelong mental health problems and has even uncovered the crucial underlying biological mechanisms—that is, the how.[11] There is a firm foundation of evidence that prenatal stress, depression, and anxiety creates the intrauterine conditions that lead to dysregulation in the offspring.[12] And our most recent research shows that when a mother has experienced early childhood adversity, not only is she more prone to prenatal depression, anxiety, and stress but also that early trauma is also linked to an altered intrauterine environment that directly impacts the baby's brain development, a process which I'll describe in more detail later on.[13]

Childhood is the second critical period in our lives.

We've known for years that infants' and children's brains change. But what has really shifted the mental health world is recognizing that our brains change throughout our whole lives. In his book *The Brain That Changes Itself*, Dr. Norman Doidge says, "Arguably the most important breakthrough in neuroscience since scientists first sketched out the brain's basic anatomy, this revolutionary discovery, called neuroplasticity, promises to overthrow the centuries-old notion that the brain is fixed and unchanging. The brain is not, as was thought, like a machine, or 'hardwired' like a computer. Neuroplasticity not only gives hope to those with mental limitations, or what was thought to be incurable brain damage, but expands our understanding of the healthy brain and the resilience of human nature."[14]

On the flip side, adversity that we experience as children has potential to rewire our brain and nervous system in a negative way, leaving us at high risk of mental health problems. Our brains are not fully developed until young adulthood, and the brain of a child relies upon healthy relationship connections and a safe, nurturing environment to grow and develop.[15] In the absence of these critical elements, children experience stress that literally changes their brain architecture and interferes with normal brain development.

Twenty-five years ago, the Adverse Childhood Experiences (ACE) Study, a milestone study of more than 8,000 people of all ages and walks of life, found that there are ten kinds of ACEs that are strongly linked to physical and mental health problems.[16] Since then, global research has identified that over 60 percent of adults have at least one ACE, with 25 percent having three or more, and discovered a staggering number of ACEs-related illnesses and biological vulnerabilities.[17] Several of these studies have demonstrated a clear association between ACEs and prenatal depression, anxiety, and stress.[18]

What does all this research mean for pregnant women? Well, we now know that mothers who have ACEs experience neurobiological dysregulation in the form of disrupted neural biomarkers, inflammation, gut microbiome changes, depression, anxiety, PTSD (post-traumatic stress disorder), and emotional dysregulation.[19, 20, 21, 22, 23, 24] Left untreated, this dysregulation continues across women's lives—and into future generations. As a group of international researchers recently notes, "Central and peripheral systems such as the brain and hypothalamic-pituitary-adrenal axis are biological conduits through which adversity can impact psychopathology across generations."[25] Infants of mothers with ACEs show increased risk of preterm birth, low birth weight, and dysregulation.[26, 27, 28]

Self-Assessment: The ACEs Questionnaire

The ACEs Questionnaire is now widely available and has been used in a growing number of countries and health systems to help people understand their risk of disease. It does cover some serious topics, so if you were in my counselling office as I share these facts, my voice would be soft and gentle, and I would look deeply into your eyes so that you felt that you were in a safe space. I would tell you that if you had a risk of diabetes because your mother and grandmother had diagnoses of diabetes, you would want to know because it would help you to put preventive strategies in your life. You would eat well, keep your BMI (body mass index) in a normal range, and you would keep your stress low. Knowing that you have an ACE is no different. We take that information, and we build a preventive plan to keep your risk low. We manage the situation. And I am here to help you through this.

To assess your ACEs risk, take a few moments to answer Yes or No to the following questions. Your ACE score is your total number of Yes responses.

YES	NO	WHILE I WAS GROWING UP, BEFORE I TURNED 18 YEARS OLD:
		1. A parent or other adult in the household would often swear at me, insult me, put me down, or humiliate me *OR* act in a way that made me afraid that I might be physically hurt.
		2. A parent or other adult in the household would often push, grab, slap, or throw something at me *OR* hit me so hard that I had marks or was injured.
		3. An adult or person at least five years older than me touched or fondled me or had me touch their body in a sexual way *OR* tried to have oral, anal, or vaginal intercourse with me.
		4. I often felt that no one in my family loved me or thought I was important or special *OR* that my family didn't look out for each other, feel close to each other, or support each other.
		5. I often felt that I didn't have enough to eat, had to wear dirty clothes, and had no one to protect me *OR* my parents were too drunk or high to take care of me or take me to the doctor if I needed it.
		6. I experienced a parental death, separation, or divorce.
		7. A household member was often pushed, grabbed, slapped, or had something thrown at him/her *OR* sometimes kicked, bitten, hit with a fist, or hit with something hard *OR* ever repeatedly hit over at least a few minutes or threatened with a gun or knife.

		8. I lived with someone who was a problem drinker or alcoholic, or who used street drugs.
		9. A household member was depressed, mentally ill, or attempted suicide.
		10. A household member went to prison.

Your Results

To put your results within the context of what we know, roughly 1 in 4 pregnant women have one to two ACEs, and 1 in 6 women have three or more. Studies show that with one or two ACEs, your chance of anxiety or depression doubles; with three or more, it triples.[29]

Why don't all women with ACEs suffer with symptoms of depression, anxiety, or stress during pregnancy? Because *all* of our experiences matter. Our relationship support, personality, level of resilience, and thinking habits (for example, optimistic and hopeful versus pessimistic) are just a few of the factors that protect and buffer us from the consequences of ACEs.

Adolescence is the third critical period in our lives.[30] During adolescence, our brains undergo a period of rapid growth and refinement. This substantial period of brain maturation creates a biological vulnerability where stressful, overwhelming situations that we face in our teen years place us at risk for the emergence of mental health problems, a main reason why certain mental health problems (such as schizophrenia, depression, anxiety) are first seen in adolescence.

Adulthood is not considered a neurobiologically critical period, but dysregulation still occurs as a result of formidable stress, hardship, and trauma. I listed several common adversities earlier in this chapter, but many of my clients are women who connected with me because they experienced situations during their pregnancy, labour, and delivery that were overwhelming and that they could not overcome. One young woman who I counselled had required an emergency caesarean section and in her anesthetic fog she heard the hospital staff talking about her prognosis. Another felt unheard and invisible before the medical staff who did not respond to concerns she expressed about her labour progress. Another faced the diagnosis of a rare congenital disorder in her unborn baby. Several others struggled with the loss of miscarriage, abortion, and stillbirth. In each case, the triggers faced during the prenatal and birthing periods dysregulated these women's nervous systems to the point where they experienced classic signs of dysregulation in the form of relentless anxiety, panic attacks, replay of memories, and poor-quality sleeps. And the research into dysregulation backs this up.[31]

As the worlds of neurobiological science and clinical work converge, the vulnerability toward mental health problems that results from dysregulation of the brain and nervous system has become the place to begin with intervention and the source of hope for those struggling with mental health problems. Re-regulating the brain and nervous system can be done with surprisingly simple techniques that, thanks to the beauty of neuroplasticity, instigate lasting change and relief when implemented as part of routine life. We'll discuss these strategies later in the book.

Genetic Vulnerability

Many women that I counsel are plagued with worry that mental health problems are a kind of genetic "birth defect" they are doomed to experience because they have a relative with some form of mental illness, but this isn't necessarily the case.

Genes are the building blocks of our DNA code, but simply

possessing a particular gene isn't enough for it to be expressed in your body. Genes can stay silent for your whole life, holding a space as part of your DNA but not really doing anything in your body. And while the Human Genome Project was expected to show revolutionary connections between genes and human disease, it did the opposite. It showed us that genes alone make very little contribution to most human traits and ailments. In fact, studies consistently show that if a mental health problem runs in your family, the chances that you'll experience it are 30 percent *at most*.[32]

Imagine a pie cut into pieces, where the entire pie represents all the possible causes of mental health problems. One-third of that pie *at most* would be genes. The remaining 70 percent of the pie would be everything else in your life—your relationships, work, home life, childhood, etc. Simply put, genes are never the total cause of illness—our experiences matter more. But knowing that a close family member (parent, sibling) has had a mental health problem alerts you to a potential biological vulnerability, and that is something you can take preventive action on.

Moreover, most health challenges with a genetic link are caused by several genes—not just one—and you have to inherit the complete package in order to develop the illness. Even then, just possessing the package of genes isn't enough. They would need to be activated by a triggering circumstance *and* then interact with absent or weakened forms of the resilience and protective factors (such as supportive relationships and good stress management) that, when strong, would otherwise push back to protect us. As you can see, genes are not deterministic, setting your fate in motion in an unrestrained, unfettered process.

Are there certain genes that have been linked to depression, anxiety, and stress? The short answer is yes. About fifteen years ago, scientists discovered genes that, in certain forms, made people more likely to react negatively to stress. They also found that people with certain genetic profiles were more likely to have their stress evolve into depression. In this case, people not only had the genes that made them more prone to stress-related depression but they were also undergoing *a lot* of stressful situations *and* their stressors were relationship oriented (such as a relationship loss versus a job loss). In other words, it was the combination of their genetic make-up and many relationship problems that increased their chances of depression.

Scientists have also found specific genes that can make us susceptible to anxiety. If you think about your own family—your brothers and sisters, father, mother, grandparents, and great-grandparents—you might be able to trace a pattern of anxiety back for a few generations. To be specific, research shows that if your mother had anxiety, you have double the risk of developing anxiety. If your mother *and* grandmother had anxiety, your risk triples.[33]

Epigenetics (the interaction between the environment and our genes) also play a role in defining our biological vulnerability and resilience. We assume that the DNA that we're born with is the DNA that we die with. But epigeneticists have discovered that certain experiences, such as ACEs, can superficially change our DNA.[34] The genes aren't permanently altered, but they are tagged with an extra molecule, and this can change what the genes do in the body. Some of the most recent research in this field shows that when women experience ACEs, their DNA gets tagged with a specific molecule (a methyl group), and their babies literally inherit the tagged DNA in areas that direct brain development, making their children more prone to mental health and developmental problems. Importantly, stressful life events that occur in adolescence or adulthood can also create epigenetic changes in certain areas of our

DNA that influence our neural regulation, stress system, and vulnerability to mental health problems.[35]

And while this sounds deterministic and unchangeable, new evidence reassures us that we can interrupt this epigenetic cycle. That epigenetic tag, like a chemical flag, can also be removed and the gene deactivated, even by simple lifestyle factors such as keeping your BMI within a normal range, regular exercise, relaxation, deep breathing, keeping stress low, and sleeping a minimum seven hours per night![36, 37] These simple lifestyle practices can help women prevent and reduce the risk of mental health problems for both themselves and their babies as evidenced by new animal research that showed that reducing stress and anxiety in pregnant rats removed the "stress and anxiety" epigenetic tags in themselves and was also passed down to the rat pups. What I love about this research is that it shows that our actions and choices can push back against the impact that negative experiences have on our genetic profiles.

Personality Vulnerabilities

Everyone has a personality type that is made up of their tendencies, preferences, and behaviours, which often becomes apparent early on in life. I raise personality here because there are two personality traits that can make a woman more prone to developing depression, anxiety, and stress: perfectionism and neuroticism.

Perfectionism

Roughly 1 in 3 women in general have unhealthy perfectionism. A few studies have called perfectionism a central reason why women develop depression, anxiety, and stress during pregnancy and at other times in their lives.[38, 39] Researchers have also found that not only is perfectionism a vulnerability for developing mental health problems but also that it maintains them.[40] In other words, perfectionism self-fuels depression, anxiety, and stress symptoms, keeping them going long-term. Anecdotally, many clinicians find that perfectionistic tendencies intensify during pregnancy and after delivery, primarily because, as one researcher who studied perfectionism in pregnant women notes, "Women with a perfectionism lifestyle try to perform their activities at an exceptional level with no errors. They maintain this behaviour in all conditions," and, I would add, at all costs.[41]

The first step is to recognize that perfectionism is a quagmire of beliefs, thoughts, and emotions that lead us to behave in the way we do—and that it can be very painful. Neuroscience would suggest that perfectionism is the rewiring of your small-child brain to fear disapproval and not meeting expectations. This manifests in three ways—and you may experience one or all of them:

1. You have unrealistic expectations of others. For example, you need others and others' work to be perfect. You need your children, partner, or friends to be and do things perfectly.
2. You believe that others have unrealistic expectations of you. You second-guess what others think of you and believe that others expect you to be perfect.
3. You have unrealistic expectations of yourself. You feel that you never make the mark, have an unrelenting inner critic, and live under a constant cloud of inadequacy.

Like most personality traits, perfectionism ranges along a spectrum from healthy to unhealthy. If you are on the healthy end of the spectrum, you set high (but realistic) standards and goals for yourself, you strive for excellence, and you're conscientious. When you don't achieve your goals, you may be disappointed but are accepting of their non-completion. You are driven by reaching your goals. On the unhealthy end of the spectrum, you may find yourself setting unrealistically high standards and goals, and when you don't attain them, you are overly critical, preoccupied with mistakes you made along the way, and excessively concerned with what you believe others think of you.[42] You are unrelenting of yourself and can't appreciate the external factors that may have interfered with meeting your goals. You are driven by a fear of failure.

For expectant mothers, perfectionism might look like a compulsion to do things perfectly from the beginning so that they don't "ruin" their unborn baby (for example, eating only healthy foods from the date of the positive pregnancy test). They feel pressure to mimic societal expectations of the "healthy and happy" pregnancy. And when they don't meet their expectations of themselves, they experience a flood of guilt and inadequacy, questioning whether they should be pregnant or if they are capable of being a "good" mother. It is these ongoing negative thoughts and feelings that are at the core of depression, anxiety, and stress—and they can be both painful and crippling. At this level, psychologists call perfectionism maladaptive; that is, it interferes with our lives and well-being.[43]

A note about the noxious effects of social media on perfectionism is warranted here. Research shows that the more time that women with high levels of perfectionism spend on social media, the greater their risk of depression and anxiety because of their tendency toward social comparison.[44] It makes sense—stories and images of gender-reveal celebrations that are timed and organized to perfection and social media posts that display idealistic photos of seemingly perfectly happy pregnant couples can contribute to a deep sense of inadequacy and pressure to perform to meet current standards of what a happy and healthy pregnancy looks like. Of course, celebratory parties and photos are not inherently bad things, but when they display an unrealistic standard, they can be damaging.

If you struggle with unhealthy perfectionism, know that you were not born like that. We believe that perfectionism emerges when children are exposed to a controlling parenting style and high, harsh performance expectations that lead us to expect and fear disapproval and disappointment of others, feel inadequate, and need to control our personal and professional lives so that mistakes are avoided.[45, 46, 47]

Neuroticism

Roughly 1 in 5 pregnant women has a neurotic personality style, making it quite common.[48] If you're like me, you cringe when you hear the words *neuroticism* or *neurotic personality*. After all, who wants to be described as neurotic? But neuroticism is simply the name of one of the "Big Five" main personality types.

If your personality tends toward neuroticism, you possess high self-awareness, carefully analyze situations, and are very conscientious. These traits make you very motivated and very good at finding solutions to challenging situations, and for this reason people with this personality type are known as the strivers.[49] And there are some very famous people that we suspect had neurotic personalities, such as Albert Einstein, Winston Churchill, and Steve Jobs.

As with all personality types, there are some aspects that we have to manage more closely. Women with a neurotic personality type have more symptoms of anxiety during pregnancy and after delivery than other personality styles—it goes with having a more reactive nature.[50] This same aspect leads them to have a significant fear of labour and delivery, greater difficulty recovering from perinatal loss (e.g., miscarriage), and puts them at a two- to threefold increase risk of postpartum anxiety and depression.[51, 52, 53, 54]

Having a neurotic personality style also makes it doubly hard for women undergoing infertility treatment, who experience the stress of treatment cycles even more intensely than do women of other personality types.

These increased risks for anxiety are linked to the experience of frequent and intense emotional reactions to stressful situations because you may struggle with controlling your emotions. For instance, you may be happy and energetic and then suddenly (in response to a situation in your life or randomly) your mood will plummet, and you'll be overcome with anxiety, worry, sadness, frustration, anger, guilt, loneliness, or fear. And there is good reason! Your negative emotions are often driven by the replay of inner, unspoken beliefs that the world is unsafe, you won't be able to manage difficulties that arise in your life, you are inadequate and don't feel like you have control over your life. For this reason, you may react to criticism in an exaggerated manner, feeling extreme guilt and replaying situations and conversations repeatedly in your mind. You may not possess all these features of neuroticism, and you may experience some more intensely than others.

Some have summarized this personality type as one that is highly sensitive to threat. Recent research highlights a genetic component.[55] From a neurobiological perspective, you may identify the features of neuroticism as signs of nervous system dysregulation. In other words, neuroticism isn't an inferior personality style. It is likely a dysregulation of the nervous system with some genetic contributions. And as with neural dysregulation, our brain and nervous system are eminently capable of re-regulating.

On a personal note, I've found that understanding my personality type has helped me to have better self-awareness about who I am and what I think and feel—that "aha" moment. And it's helped me to appreciate the strengths and areas for growth that all personality types offer. While a neurotic personality style does mean that you're more inclined to be reactive to stress and emotions, and more vulnerable to anxiety, you can learn to successfully manage your thoughts and emotions to lower your risk of anxiety and help you to have an emotionally healthy pregnancy.

By treating neuroticism as not just personality (a set of traits and behaviours) but also as neurobiological dysregulation, pregnant women may reduce the risk it plays in prenatal depression, anxiety, or stress. I'll touch on how to do this by implementing bottom-up techniques (body to brain) in later chapters. These can all move you toward a more positive, even emotional experience that is based on safety rather than threat.

When we think about biological vulnerabilities, remember that the root words of vulnerability are *vulnus* and *vulnerare*, which mean "wound" and "to wound," respectively. Biological vulnerability is like that inner wound—a hurt or an injury that has come to us largely through generational and early influences. There are two key insights that stem from this reflection.

First, wounds can be healed. We are not at the fate of our biology. While past experiences beyond our control may have contributed to our vulnerability, the wonder of neuroplasticity (our brain's ability to change) assures us that our present-day experiences can also affect biological changes—and healing can happen.

Second, biological vulnerabilities are not your fault. This is something I often say to my clients, and I am saying it to you now. It isn't your fault. You didn't do anything to suffer as you have. You didn't do anything to your unborn baby. There are complex, intergenerational forces that come together to produce mental health struggles. But these cycles can be broken.[56] And sometimes that is the role of tough times and difficult experiences—to help us to heal ourselves and future generations.

Risk Factors of Mental Health Problems in Pregnancy

Many women worry that developing mental health problems in pregnancy (and postpartum) is the result of some cruel, random process. However, there are well-defined risk factors that, when combined with an underlying biological vulnerability, *can* result in an episode of depression, anxiety, or stress.

From years of research, our team has found that four experiences have the greatest risk for prenatal depression, anxiety, and stress: relationship trouble, toxic stress in the year before pregnancy, a history of mental health problems, and lack of support. Again, these can be tied to dysregulation as each of these risk factors relates to feeling unsafe. Studies conducted in developed countries such as Canada, the US, Australia, and Great Britain and in developing countries such as Indonesia, Pakistan, and Africa have found that these risk factors are common across women of all ages, economic cultures, races, and countries.

Relationship Trouble

Relationship trouble, such as having an unsupportive (both emotionally and practically) or uninterested partner, experiencing a pattern of frequent conflict, or being dissatisfied with your relationship have been shown consistently to elevate your risk of depression, anxiety, and stress two to five times. Some studies show that as many as 40 percent of pregnant women with anxiety feel that they have inadequate partner support (four times that of women without mental health symptoms), and almost 60 percent report having tension in their partner relationship (twice that of women without mental health symptoms). And it's not just pregnant women who are affected. Relationship troubles also affect partners, increasing their risk of psychological distress.[57]

Toxic Stress

Toxic stress is common, with as many as 80 percent of pregnant women reporting moderate or high levels of stress.[58] Many studies show that stressful experiences that trigger depression and anxiety and can range from mild experiences to very difficult life situations, such as you or your partner losing a job, experiencing a relationship breakdown, or losing a loved one. The higher your perceived stress—how much stress you feel and internalize amid life circumstances—the greater your risk of mental health symptoms, increasing your risk three- to five-fold.[59]

History of Mental Health Problems

Having a previous mental health problem is the strongest predictor of experiencing depression, anxiety, and stress during pregnancy.[60, 61] Research shows that if you've experienced anxiety or depression before you became pregnant (including as a child or teen), you are six to eleven times more likely to develop depression during pregnancy. When practitioners gather health history, they commonly ask the three general questions. If you're concerned about having this risk factor, take a moment to answer the questions on the following pages.

Your Emotional Health History

Simply respond with Yes or No, and then give yourself 1 point for each Yes.

- I have had a bout of depression or anxiety that lasted two weeks or more at some time in the past.
- I have experienced depression or anxiety with a previous pregnancy or after delivery.
- My mother, father, or a sibling has experienced (or been diagnosed with) depression, anxiety, or another mental health problem.

Your Results

If you scored 0, you have no personal or family history of depression or anxiety, so your risk is low. The higher your score, the greater the impact of your personal and family history becoming a risk factor for depression or anxiety during pregnancy or after you have your baby. Having a previous episode of depression, anxiety, and stress may signal the need to invest time and effort in neuro-regulating strategies, such as the BEE Protocol in Chapter 7.

Lack of Support

A lack of support, such as not having a trusted friend or group of friends, almost triples the risk of depression, anxiety, and stress.[62]

And this makes sense, because new neurobiological research reveals that when we are connected to others in a safe relationship, our autonomic nervous system is calmed and regulated. As a neonatal nurse, I would often put a newborn baby on their mother's bare chest and then notice on the electronic monitors the slowing and regulating of the baby's heart and respiratory rates. I was amazed to learn that the same principle applies to adults! In fact, in my counselling practice, I would sometimes give couples a homework assignment to hug once per day for two minutes because the simple act of hugging engenders physiological co-regulation—and trust. Because low support can be so detrimental, and strong support so resiliency enhancing, I invite you to complete the Maternity Social Support Scale as a check-in on your social support.

SELF-ASSESSMENT

The Maternity Social Support Scale[63]

The following six questions ask about the quality of your relationship with your partner and close friends to help you assess the degree of social support you currently have. You can fill this out any time, but ideally at least once during your pregnancy and again within the first few months after delivery. Life will change dramatically after you have your baby, and it's a good idea to check in and identify whether your level of support continues to meet your needs.

Answer each of the questions with one of the five responses: always, most of the time, some of the time, rarely, and never. Then add up the responses for your total score.

For each of the following statements, please tick the box which shows how you feel about the support you have right now:

A. I have good friends who support me.

Always	Most of the time	Some of the time	Rarely	Never
5	4	3	2	1

B. My family is always there for me.

Always	Most of the time	Some of the time	Rarely	Never
5	4	3	2	1

C. My husband/partner helps me a lot.

Always	Most of the time	Some of the time	Rarely	Never
5	4	3	2	1

D. There is conflict with my husband/partner.

Always	Most of the time	Some of the time	Rarely	Never
1	2	3	4	5

E. I feel controlled by my husband/partner.

Always	Most of the time	Some of the time	Rarely	Never
1	2	3	4	5

F. I feel loved by my husband/partner.

Always	Most of the time	Some of the time	Rarely	Never
5	4	3	2	1

Your Results

YOUR SCORE	THE MEANING OF YOUR SCORE	YOUR NEXT STEPS
6–18	Low social support	Overall, you feel you don't have enough social support, which may be difficult for you as you move through pregnancy and into parenthood.
19–24	Medium social support	Overall, you have medium social support. Your relationships with your friends, family, and partner offer some emotional and practical support, but you may feel at times that you could use more.
25–30	Adequate social support	Overall, you have adequate support. Most of the time, you feel that your relationships are supportive and that you are well-prepared for your transition.

Questions A and B focus on the support of your friends and family. If you scored 3 or below on these questions, you likely lack strong support from this circle. Relationships are two-sided, and one person can't improve the relationship as much as they may desire to. Consider whether there is anything you can do to build those relationships.

Questions C, D, E, and F focus on the quality of your relationship with your partner. If you scored between 1 and 2, consider seeking support for you and your partner, such as individual or couples' counselling. If you scored 3, you and your partner may want to seek outside help, or you can use the strategies in the following section on pushback factors to strengthen your relationship so that it's mutually satisfying and supportive.

Other Risk Factors

Much work in the past decade has focused on the link between our attachment pattern (how we relate to others and expect others to respond to us) and mental health. In pregnancy and postpartum, we are interested in two sides: a mother's own early attachment patterns and her attachment to her baby.

Our attachment pattern is formed when we're young and follows us into adulthood, framing the way that we view and act in relationships and how we tend to cope with stressors in our lives. The two broad kinds of attachment are insecure and secure attachment.

Someone with a secure attachment pattern will reach out to their partner or a close friend or family member for comfort and support in times of difficulty and naturally expect (and trust) that they'll be available and willing to help.[64] They'll have a natural ease and trust in their relationships, feel comfortable being alone, and be able to manage conflict and relationship troubles.

Conversely, when someone with an insecure attachment reaches out for help, they'll want excessive closeness, seek continual reassurance, and fear that the person won't be able to give them what they need. They may find it hard to trust people and are generally wary in relationships—both in what they give and receive. They often feel insecure being alone because their self-worth comes primarily from their relationships. Studies show that people with insecure attachment tend to have disrupted stress systems and so are more physically and emotionally taxed under stress.[65]

As I see that fact on the page in black and white, it seems like a massive understatement, because we now suspect that the disrupted stress system didn't begin at the macro level of the brain and nervous system—it began at the cellular level with the more than one hundred thousand sensory proteins on every body cell that read our environment for danger.[66] Because the trajectory of these embryonic cells sets the foundation of growth of our entire body, it's critically important for the cells of the embryo to grow in a uterine environment that is flooded with nurturing goodness stemming from a mother at low stress, threat, and danger. When those cells grow in a toxic environment, the embryo's sense of safety and trust is disrupted, and new thinking is that insecure attachment begins at this early, cellular level. The good news is that we can shift these early effects, and the first step is to recognize when we are dysregulated.

There are other, less common and lower risk factors for prenatal depression, anxiety, and stress, such as infertility treatment. Between 10 percent to 14 percent of women who have undergone infertility treatment experience depression, anxiety, or stress in pregnancy.[67] However, most studies, ours included, show that they rarely continue into pregnancy unless women have other risk factors, such as partner conflict.[68]

Other studies have shown that about 16 percent to 22 percent of women who had a pregnancy loss experience depression, anxiety, or stress post-loss and are at increased risk for mental health problems in subsequent pregnancies.[69, 70] One study from Denmark reported that 41 percent of women who had a previous pregnancy loss experienced high stress compared to 23 percent of pregnant women who never had a loss.[71] Pregnant women who are hospitalized for high-risk pregnancies tend to have higher rates and greater severity of depression (20 percent) and anxiety (39 percent).[72, 73]

Having risk factors for mental illness isn't good or bad. It's part of the fabric of your life—your story. While you can change some of these, you can't change all of them. That's why it's important to build your emotional health, which we'll discuss throughout the book, so that you have a line of defense when difficult things happen in life. You can also lower your risk and even prevent depression, anxiety, and stress with pushback factors.

Pushback Factors for Mental Health Problems in Pregnancy

As always, there is hope to be found in what can be difficult facts. Significant risk factors, such as our relationship with our partner, tell us that there is something about those experiences that are critical for our well-being. When we have their negative aspects (such as partner conflict), they are risks.[74] When we have their positive aspects (such as partner support), they are strengths. The four risk factors that I've discussed—partner troubles, experiencing stress, having had a mental health problem in the past, and inadequate social support—are, when strengthened, the greatest source of resilience you can possess. They can act as pushback factors because they can reduce our risk of depression, anxiety, and stress.

For example, if you are having a year filled with stressful life events—your mother was taken seriously ill, you lost your job and are experiencing financial difficulties, and you were just diagnosed with gestational diabetes—this accumulation of stressful life events can increase your risk for developing depression and anxiety. However, if your partner relationship was intimate, low-conflict, and supportive, your risk may decrease, and your resilience can increase.[75]

On a neurobiological level, pushback factors are anything that lower your risk for depression, anxiety, and stress because they maintain the nervous system in a regulated state. Those identified in the prenatal mental health and mental health literature in general include spending time in nature; play (e.g., sports, movies, reading); supportive relationships; feeling connected; restful sleep; exercise; hope, optimism; resiliency; and positive childhood experiences. In this chapter, I'd like to specifically focus on resilience, coping strategies, and social support.

Resilience

The research definition of resilience is the group of biological, psychological, social, and cultural factors that determine how we respond to a stressful situation.[76] But neuroscience might define it as a well-regulated brain and nervous system that quickly re-regulates within the context of difficult life circumstances. As a pushback factor, resilience helps us to function in the face of debilitating stress.

Resilience isn't borne out of an easy life with no challenges. In fact, there is a phenomenon called the Steeling Effect, which shows that people who experience *some* adversity in their lives have better mental health and are more satisfied with their lives than are people with either *a lot* of adversity or *no* adversity. In other words, too much stress or stress that lasts too long wears us down, and our resilience suffers. Too little stress doesn't give us enough experience and practice dealing with adversity to build up our capacity to handle it in a good way. And *some* adversity is good because it makes us more resilient.

Tolerance to adversity is rooted in neuroplasticity. While significant adversity, such as multiple ACEs, can take our nervous system off-line so that it cannot re-regulate easily on its own, research by neuroscientist and pioneering stress researcher Dr. Bruce McEwen suggests that our brain actually *adapts* to moderate stress, causing our brain and nervous system to change and grow and promote regulation, or resilience.[77]

How does this show up in your life? With greater resilience, you adapt to challenging situations more readily. A situation arises, your brain and nervous system become activated, and then it settles quickly, and you engage in clear-thinking problem solving. This helps build confidence about your ability to handle change and stress so that uncertainty about life situations and future outcomes is less daunting. With this, the experience stimulates *more* neuroplasticity, forming healthy brain networks that help to increase your resilience even more. And our research shows that resilient mothers have resilient children.[78]

SELF-ASSESSMENT

The Brief Resilience Scale[79]

The following assessment measures your ability to bounce back when faced with challenges in the past month. You can use it any time, but ideally at least once during your pregnancy and again after you have your baby.

Answer each question with one of the five responses, add up your scores, then divide your total score by 6. For example, if your total score to the six questions was 17, you would divide 17 by 6 to get a final score of 2.83.

I tend to bounce back quickly after hard times.

Strongly disagree	Disagree	Neutral	Agree	Strongly agree
1	2	3	4	5

I have a hard time making it through stressful events.

Strongly disagree	Disagree	Neutral	Agree	Strongly agree
5	4	3	2	1

It does not take me long to recover from a stressful event.

Strongly disagree	Disagree	Neutral	Agree	Strongly agree
1	2	3	4	5

It is hard for me to snap back when something bad happens.

Strongly disagree	Disagree	Neutral	Agree	Strongly agree
5	4	3	2	1

I usually come through difficult times with little trouble.

Strongly disagree	Disagree	Neutral	Agree	Strongly agree
1	2	3	4	5

I tend to take a long time to get over setbacks in my life.

Strongly disagree	Disagree	Neutral	Agree	Strongly agree
5	4	3	2	1

Total Score	
Divided by 6	

Your Results

YOUR SCORE	THE MEANING OF YOUR SCORE
1.00–2.99	Low resilience
3.00–4.30	Normal resilience
4.31–5.00	High resilience

If you discovered that your resilience is on the low side, it's not because you don't have the ability to manage life's tough situations. Your score reflects a dysregulated nervous system that has probably been jarred by one or more significant challenges in your life, including being worn down by chronic stress, having symptoms of depression or anxiety that make it difficult for you to cope with problems, or not having had the opportunity to build helpful coping strategies. Later in the book, we'll discuss the ways you can improve your resilience to enhance your ability to cope with and recover from stressful situations and make it easier to manage—and enjoy—your transition to parenthood.

Coping Strategies

Coping strategies are cognitive and behavioural efforts to manage specific external and/or internal demands that tax or exceed the resources of the person.[80, 81] For instance, walking in nature or deep breathing are behavioural coping strategies—actions you take—to reduce your distress.

The most effective coping strategies are behavioural, since they target neural regulation, moving you from the dysregulation to regulation.[82] While cognitive strategies target our thoughts, behavioural strategies operate on a bottom-up, body-to-brain framework of regulating the neural system first so that the positive effects flow to the body (our heart rate slows, we breathe more easily, our tummy settles down, our shoulders relax).

The goal of all coping strategies is to reduce your distress; but coping strategies that first and foremost target neural regulation also promote neuroplasticity so that the effect of the strategy is long-lasting and not time limited to just while it's being done. For example, although we've long observed that exercise reduces depression, a review of all research done over the past twenty years revealed that the reason exercise works is because it increases a chemical called brain-derived neurotrophic factor (BDNF), which enhances brain neuroplasticity (e.g., healthy neuronal growth).[83]

Social Support

Years of research show that social support—having a trusted, supportive other—is one of the strongest defenses against depression, anxiety, and stress. As humans, we're wired for relationship. When we experience difficult times, we have an innate need to share our experience with others to feel understood and less alone. We need an injection of hope and promise from others' experiences facing and overcoming similar difficulties. And we need compassion and empathy from others. In fact, new research shows that our brain registers social pain (interpersonal loss, conflict, being excluded) in the same way that it registers physical pain, which is why not having social support feels painful.[84, 85]

The term *social support* doesn't convey the critical feature of safety that is foundational for our brain and nervous system to calm and re-regulate in the presence of relationship, but there are vast neurological benefits of a safe relationship. The feeling of not being alone that floods us in the presence of another who shares in our experience is the emotional manifestation of neurobiological regulation. This is why well-meaning partners who offer to unload the dishwasher when we are feeling high stress doesn't quite cut it from a supportive standpoint! I share that scenario because in our long marriage of over thirty-five years, this was my husband's early response. He thought he was being helpful, reducing a workload burden. But I remember saying to him, "I just need to know it's going to be okay." It was my callout for safety. And then he would hold me and say, "It's going to be okay." So, he needed a little direction, and that's okay, too.

The Consequences of Depression, Anxiety, and Stress in Pregnancy

Why do mental health problems in pregnancy matter? Why is it important to know the causes, risk factors, and pushback strategies? Because it motivates us to make our mental health care system better for women and babies. And because the pain, guilt, and regret of not knowing and wishing they had done things differently plagues far too many women. In my experience, women don't want to be short-changed by having only select facts. They want the full story.

Research has found that prenatal depression, anxiety, stress, and ACEs can restructure or reprogram the baby's brain and nervous system through a process called fetal programming.[86] Fetal programming was discovered through the work of scientist Dr. David Barker who in 2004 studied how poor nutrition during pregnancy might be linked to heart disease in the infant, and now it's an entire branch of science on its own: developmental origins of health and disease. Today, we understand that the prenatal environment has the potential to rewire the unborn baby's brain and body systems so that they are more prone to a mental health problem, and this rewiring can begin when the fertilized egg is only days old.[87, 88]

Ultimately, fetal programming occurs in an environment of threat and lack of safety. When the uterine environment is sub-optimal (e.g., due to stress, insufficient nutrients, inflammation), the baby's systems interpret it as a dangerous, threatening environment, and the development of the brain and body systems wiring is reprogrammed to build architecture for survival, often jarring their nervous system into dysregulation.[89] And ours and other research shows that it isn't just severe depression, anxiety, or stress that has this effect—a fetus can have an increased risk when the mother has sub-clinical symptoms that are barely detectible, which is why it's so important to be in tune with your mental health.[90]

A recent groundbreaking study also showed that this dysregulation isn't just passed down from mother to child—it can start generations earlier; dysregulation effectively walks down through the lineage.[91] In other words, it can be a vicious cycle, with the mother having a biological vulnerability for mental health problems because of her own fetal programming.

One way the fetus' body is reprogrammed is through epigenetic changes.[92] As previously noted, our genes are like small command centres that direct activities in our body and when we face a threat, an extra molecule can attach to affected genes and change what it does in the body. For instance, if the gene affected directs stress responsiveness, the extra molecule might amp up activity so that we are more reactive to stress. These aren't permanent changes to our genes but *early* epigenetic changes can instigate long-term changes in brain and body organ structure that can carry on into adulthood in the form of predisposition to depression, anxiety, stress, and other mental and physical health problems.[93]

In the field of perinatal mental health, we've learned that women who have experienced ACEs have epigenetic tags on some of their genes, and these tagged genes are inherited by the child.[94] (Historically, we suspected that the reason children experienced dysregulation and other effects of a mother's childhood adversity was because of suboptimal parenting patterns; for example, the mother was unable to parent well because of her own childhood experiences). But now we know that epigenetics play a role.

There is another underlying biological reason for a woman's early adversity affecting her child. Almost a decade ago, a landmark study found that when a mother had experienced childhood trauma, high levels of her stress hormones would flow across the placenta and into the baby's bloodstream through the maternalfetal circulatory network.[95] Normally, the placenta contains an enzyme that, when the mother's blood flows through it, inactivates the stress chemicals, kind of like a water filter that takes out impurities.[96, 97] But when mothers have experienced early adversity, this placental enzyme doesn't work properly, and the stress chemicals flow through to the baby's blood and amniotic fluid. And once the baby's brain is flooded with stress chemicals, it rewires and reconfigures to adapt to what it perceives as a dangerous environment—effectively reprogramming the baby's brain and nervous system in a way that reflects intergenerational transmission of adversity. The study suggests that the medical community needs to better understand the biological pathways of adversity to develop effective interventions. This is precisely the goal of this book—to optimize the brain health of mother and baby.

Dysregulation in Infants and Children

In infants, dysregulation shows up as persistent crying, sleeping problems, feeding challenges, and being difficult to soothe and settle from 6 months to 2.5 years.[98] In children, neural dysregulation is a combination of emotional, behavioural, and attentional problems seen between 4 and 9.5 years of age, which, in and of themselves, place the child at increased risk of mental health problems, such as depression, anxiety, autism spectrum disorders, and attention and hyperactivity disorders. [99, 100, 101, 102, 103, 104]

But not all children of women with prenatal depression, anxiety, and stress show signs of dysregulation.

First, roughly 15 percent to 20 percent of children whose mothers have prenatal symptoms experience clinical signs of dysregulation as I have described above.[105, 106] But I would like to add a caveat. Most studies assess for children for obvious signs of dysregulation. It is possible for children to be dysregulated and not show such overt signs. I mention this because I know you want the very best for your child and because we now know how to help children re-regulate their nervous system. Global research and clinical work are showing some very hopeful solutions for helping children to re-regulate their nervous system, such as Safe and Sound Protocol and Tomatis Therapy discussed in Chapter 7.

Second, the best evidence we have today shows that the risk of children experiencing difficulties increases when a woman experiences *chronic* depression, anxiety, or stress, or long-standing dysregulation.[107, 108] The risk factors that contribute to chronic depression, anxiety, and stress are having significant, ongoing partner conflict; a combination of depression, anxiety, and/or stress; a history of depression; few social supports; childhood adversity;

persistent poor sleep quality; and using antidepressants before or during pregnancy. But not everyone carries these risks.

I can't end this chapter without also giving you hope. Now that we know that dysregulation plays such a major role in your and your child's well-being, we can use that to our advantage, targeting intervention at re-regulation. Here is a preview of strategies that you can use to regulate your new baby's brain:

- Hold your baby. The simple act of holding your baby changes their brain, making it healthier and reversing some of the genetic changes that may have occurred before birth.
- Maintain a strong partner relationship where you both feel satisfied with your relationship. This co-regulation helps you and your partner be regulated, which helps your baby to regulate their brain and nervous system, too.
- Attend to your child's needs with sensitivity, such as soothing your child when they are distressed. This helps your child to feel safe and secure, which is foundational for healthy brain development.
- Talk to your child while you are doing other things.
- Interact with your child, keeping eye contact with them when you are talking to them.
- Read to your child.
- Play with your child.[109]

In the world of perinatal mental health, we have chopped up the perinatal period into phases—before pregnancy, during pregnancy (prenatal), after pregnancy (postpartum)—but this approach hasn't allowed us to see the full breadth of the story of women's lives. For instance, years of research has shown us that the largest risk factor for prenatal mental health problems is having had depression, anxiety, or toxic stress in the past. We know that the proportion of women who develop depression or anxiety for the first time in pregnancy is low—somewhere between 2 percent and 30 percent, which means that more than 70 percent have experienced symptoms at some point earlier in their lives.[110] The biggest risk factor for *postpartum* depression and anxiety is *prenatal* depression and anxiety. Many women continue to experience symptoms long after their baby is born—our research shows rates of 35 percent continuation of symptoms from pregnancy to 11 years postpartum, and other studies from Canada, France, and Australia report rates as high as 50 percent over a period of up to 20 years.[111, 112] All these studies conclude that there is a stable pattern of mental health from pregnancy to postpartum: without intervention, symptoms of depression, anxiety, and stress generally stay at the same level across and beyond the perinatal period.[113, 114, 115, 116]

Looking at these data, I suggest that what we are seeing in perinatal mental health is part of a pattern of *long-term brain and nervous system dysregulation*. Pre-pregnancy mental health problems aren't just a "risk" for prenatal depression, anxiety, and stress. Prenatal mental health problems aren't just a "risk" for postpartum depression and anxiety. And prenatal and postnatal mental health problems aren't just a "risk" for chronic, long-standing depression and anxiety. Rather, they tell the story of long-term neural dysregulation. And in this book, I will teach you how you can disrupt this lifelong trajectory—starting with the foundations of good mental health.

CHAPTER 2

The Foundations of Good Mental Health

Before we jump into specific mental health concerns during pregnancy, we need to understand what mental health and mental illness are. So, what is mental health? For a long time, we defined mental health as the absence of mental illness, and as practitioners, our goal was to treat a person's *symptoms* of depression, anxiety, and stress. However, research shows us that 2 out of 3 people with such symptoms also have clear signs of mental health such as the ability to bounce back from challenges (resilience or resiliency), accept their circumstances (acceptance), and problem-solve their next steps. In other words, mental health and mental illness occupy the same continuum. From this work, we've learned that improving mental health isn't just about lessening people's distress by reducing symptoms of depression, anxiety, or stress; it also involves developing the markers of good mental health (like the ability to exercise choice and set boundaries).

Recent neuroscience research has shifted how we understand mental health and mental illness, which in turn is leading to a shift in how we treat mental illness. For decades, our sole focus was top-down: often addressing symptoms with cognitive-based therapies that help change our thinking and perspectives, which in turn changes our behaviour and fosters the growth of skills. The new paradigm of mental health led by neuroscientists, trauma researchers, and clinicians introduces a treatment approach for mental illness that is bottom-up; i.e., it starts with the brain and nervous system as the cause of the symptoms. In a recent academic paper, psychologist and neuroscientist Dr. Stephen Porges writes, "Contemporary strategies for health and well-being fail our biological needs by not acknowledging that feelings of safety emerge from internal physiological states regulated by the autonomic nervous system."[1] That is, good mental health begins with the foundation of a regulated brain and nervous system; mental health problems occur when our nervous system becomes dysregulated. This shift toward a neurobiological understanding and treatment of mental illness is so dramatic that it is prompting some to reframe mental health as brain health and treatment as healing.[2, 3]

Does this mean that everything we ever thought about good mental health is incorrect? Absolutely not! Think of our burgeoning understanding of mental health as the layers of an archeological dig. When archeologists brush away the top layer of soil, they find certain relics. As they dig, they continue to discover relics, which together paint a picture of what happened at that particular site. Deeper layers expose even more foundational insights about the culture and nature of the peoples or animals in that region.

Scientific research and clinical wisdom allow us to dig more deeply into the nature of a problem and understand the foundations of the illness more completely so we can better treat illness. Let me emphasize that for decades, the research and practice of top-down mental health care (therapies like cognitive behaviour therapy) helped many people and was effective—to a degree. But as our understanding of mental health expanded to focus on brain health—the area of neuroscience—we now know that the *most* effective approach is a bottom-up one that *begins* with the health of the brain and nervous system. Rather than simply reducing symptoms, advanced neuroscientific treatment techniques allow us to restore and heal the brain and nervous system for quicker and longer-lasting results.[4] And these simple strategies are taking their place as a central part of effective mental health care, which is immensely good news for anyone whose mental health is suffering.

In this chapter, I'll discuss the foundations of good mental health from the perspective of the new neuroscience paradigm and share simple top-down and bottom-up techniques and strategies that you can use to regulate your nervous system so that you can achieve and maintain good mental health. These are techniques that we all should use regularly, for none of us is untouched by life challenges that are capable of jarring our nervous system into dysregulation.

Good Mental Health: A Neuroscience Perspective

What is good mental health? You may be expecting me to begin with a statement like, "It is the feeling of inner calm and peace—the absence of tension and turmoil." We could all agree that these feelings would signal a sense of well-being. However, these felt markers of emotional well-being have their roots in a regulated nervous system.

Our brain and nervous system are regulated when we feel physically and emotionally safe. Psychologist and neuroscientist Dr. Stephen Porges describes it this way: "Feeling safe functions as a subjective index of a neural platform that supports both sociality and the homeostatic processes optimizing health, growth, and restoration . . . feeling safe is our subjective interpretation of internal bodily feelings that are being conveyed via bi-directional neural pathways between our bodily organs and our brain . . . the cues of safety."[5] And when we feel safe, our body functions optimally. The signs of good mental health are the signs of a regulated nervous system. You experience:

- optimal health and performance
- calm
- trust and connection with others
- high levels of problem solving
- curiosity and creativity
- compassion and openness toward others
- focus and attention
- energy
- joy and happiness
- a sense of being grounded, fun, and peaceful[6]

In her book *The Polyvagal Theory in Therapy*, psychologist Deb Dana notes that our lives reflect our regulated state in that we are organized, we follow through with plans, exercise self-care, enjoy play time, do things with and for others, feel productive at work, and have a general sense of being together and regulated. She describes the health effects of this regulated state as a heathy heart, normal blood pressure, healthy immune system, good digestion, restful sleep, and a general feeling of well-being.[7]

Ask yourself this question: How safe do you feel at this moment on a scale of 1 to 10, with 1 being not safe at all and 10 being completely safe? Don't overthink the question—the number that pops into your head is the one to pay attention to. How is it possible to be in the comfort of your own home or sitting in a lovely, inviting coffee shop reading this book and feel that there is some threat lurking—something that makes your stomach go into knots, your shoulders tighten, your breathing and heartbeat quicken, and your neck tense?

Why do so many of us feel unsafe much of the time, living our lives in a heightened state of fear, anxiety, and worry as if we were anticipating a lion to jump out from behind every tree we pass? In his book *Why Zebras Don't Get Ulcers*, Dr. Robert Sapolsky notes that while we do face mortal danger at times (e.g., traffic accidents, natural disasters), the threats and dangers of modern society are often social in nature. [8] In other words, our sense of unsafety comes from our relationships.

In what he dubs the SCARF model, Dr. David Rock describes five situations that the brain interprets as threat: Status (our relative importance to others), Certainty (our ability to predict the future), Autonomy (our sense of control in and over our lives/ events), Relatedness (how safe we feel with others), and Fairness (how fair we see our exchanges with others).[9] Notice that none of these are imminent physical dangers. No, the threats of modern-day society are more subtle and highly relational. Our brain detects threat when we perceive ourselves as less important than others, feel uncertain, don't feel we have control over our circumstances, don't feel safe with others, and perceive that we have not been treated fairly or have been betrayed. And when the brain detects threat, the host of reactions that form the stress response ensue, and we show the physical, emotional, and cognitive signs of dysregulation that I shared earlier. In a regulated nervous system, that stress response from start to finish lasts but a few seconds. In a dysregulated nervous system, it can last for days, weeks, or even years.

Research over the past twenty years has revealed several markers of mental health: self-awareness, emotional regulation, self-acceptance, trusting relationships, healthy coping skills, sense of purpose, growth mindset, autonomy, flexibility, self-control, and positive emotions. These markers of mental health are good indicators of a regulated nervous system. When our brain and nervous system are dysregulated, these expressions of a regulated nervous system will be quieter in our lives. When regulated, they will be amplified, and we will feel at our best.

SELF-ASSESSMENT

The Brain and Nervous System Regulation Questionnaire

I suggest completing this five-minute check-in any time you want to assess your brain and nervous system regulation. As you learn to read your body and understand signals of dysregulation, you'll find less need to complete a formal assessment. The goal of this assessment is to train yourself to know when your brain and nervous system are dysregulated, and then to employ techniques to bring your nervous system back to a regulated state. Like taking your temperature when you are ill as an indicator of an underlying process and how your body is responding to it, these markers help you to understand the underlying state of your nervous system.

For each statement, select one of the six responses to indicate how much you agree or disagree with it, then add up the score of each of the eighteen questions to identify how regulated your brain and nervous system are.

MARKER	QUESTION

Self-awareness — I have a clear sense of my values, purpose, strengths, limitations, boundaries, and triggers.

Strongly disagree	Somewhat disagree	Somewhat agree	Strongly agree
1	2	3	4

Sense of calm and peace — I have a strong sense of calm and peace.

Strongly disagree	Somewhat disagree	Somewhat agree	Strongly agree
1	2	3	4

Curiosity — I am curious and interested.

Strongly disagree	Somewhat disagree	Somewhat agree	Strongly agree
1	2	3	4

Creativity — I have a strong sense of creativity, thinking up new ideas, strategies, and ways of doing things.

Strongly disagree	Somewhat disagree	Somewhat agree	Strongly agree
1	2	3	4

Joy — I have a quiet sense of joy and find it easy to laugh and play freely.

Strongly disagree	Somewhat disagree	Somewhat agree	Strongly agree
1	2	3	4

Emotional regulation — I manage my emotions easily.

Strongly disagree	Somewhat disagree	Somewhat agree	Strongly agree
1	2	3	4

Self-acceptance I accept my strengths and am realistic about my limitations.

Strongly disagree	Somewhat disagree	Somewhat agree	Strongly agree
1	2	3	4

Trusting relationships I feel connected to my significant others. I trust my significant others.

Strongly disagree	Somewhat disagree	Somewhat agree	Strongly agree
1	2	3	4

Social connectedness I feel socially connected to others.

Strongly disagree	Somewhat disagree	Somewhat agree	Strongly agree
1	2	3	4

Protectiveness I don't feel the need to protect myself from others.

Strongly disagree	Somewhat disagree	Somewhat agree	Strongly agree
1	2	3	4

Sense of psychological safety I feel a strong sense of safety where I feel cared for, respected, and heard by others.

Strongly disagree	Somewhat disagree	Somewhat agree	Strongly agree
1	2	3	4

Healthy coping skills I have strategies that I use to cope when life becomes stressful or challenging.

Strongly disagree	Somewhat disagree	Somewhat agree	Strongly agree
1	2	3	4

Sense of purpose

I have a strong sense of purpose and direction in my life, which I work out through creating and accomplishing goals. I feel productive in my life's work.

Strongly disagree	Somewhat disagree	Somewhat agree	Strongly agree
1	2	3	4

Growth mindset

I believe that growing and developing is important and take opportunities to develop my skills and talents.

Strongly disagree	Somewhat disagree	Somewhat agree	Strongly agree
1	2	3	4

Autonomy

I live by my values, unaffected by the pressures and unfounded expectations of others; I set clear and reasonable boundaries. I feel free to make choices that are best in line with my values and priorities.

Strongly disagree	Somewhat disagree	Somewhat agree	Strongly agree
1	2	3	4

Flexibility

I accept reality and exercise flexibility and resilience rather than fighting against my circumstances or feeling trapped.

Strongly disagree	Somewhat disagree	Somewhat agree	Strongly agree
1	2	3	4

Self-control

I feel in control of my life where I feel able to make changes as I need.

Strongly disagree	Somewhat disagree	Somewhat agree	Strongly agree
1	2	3	4

Positive emotions   I experience positive emotions; I also experience and accept my negative emotions.

Strongly disagree	Somewhat disagree	Somewhat agree	Strongly agree
1	2	3	4

Your Results

The higher your score, the more regulated your brain and nervous system are, and therefore, the greater your mental health. You don't have to score high in all the markers of mental health to be flourishing. The markers where you indicated that you somewhat or strongly disagree are specific areas that will benefit from development and the research-based strategies outlined below. Remember: change happens with small, consistent steps. Start with implementing one strategy in your life before you consider adding another.

Self-awareness

Some would say that self-awareness is the first step toward building emotional health because out of self-awareness comes choice. Self-awareness is about understanding the patterns that make up you—your core values, purpose, strengths, limitations, triggers and reactions, boundaries, priorities, etc.—and how your behaviour affects others.

When our nervous system has been chronically dysregulated, especially due to early trauma, we grow up being unaware of ourselves. In *Transforming the Living Legacy of Trauma*, Dr. Janina Fisher calls this a *loss of who we are*. We grow up not knowing who we are, what we like and dislike, what our needs, values, and priorities are. We may defer to others' preferences or see others' ideas and needs as more important than our own and be unable to set healthy boundaries.

Here are five top-down strategies that will also enhance your self-awareness:

1. *The 5-second daily pause.* Stop periodically during the day for 5 seconds to close your eyes, breathe, and simply identify what you are feeling in that moment. Ask yourself: What is the emotion I am experiencing? What thoughts do I have? What do I feel in my body?
2. *Journaling.* If writing helps you to clarify your thoughts and feelings, then journaling regularly can help you to find patterns in your triggers, reactions, and feelings.
3. *Connecting.* Debriefing with a trusted friend on how you're feeling, putting words to feelings, is also valuable.
4. *Emotion cards.* Most are decks of cards with a single emotion on each one. You can scan the deck and pick out the emotions that resonate with how you're feeling in that moment. We use them for children, but the adult versions are immensely helpful if you struggle to put words to how you are feeling.
5. *Counselling.* Excellent therapists can help you identify and validate your feelings.

Sense of Calm and Peace, Curiosity, Creativity, Joy

I've grouped these indicators of brain and nervous system regulation together because they stem from the same root—feeling safe. Think about the last time that you experienced calm and peace, or a sense of quiet joy. Hold that picture in your mind and allow yourself to remember what you saw, smelled, heard, and felt.

For me, it was late evening, and I was doing a final check of my sheep and their lambs on our sheep farm. We were in a beautiful pasture, dotted with white daisies and yellow buttercups and long grass that was flowing gently in the wind. The light breeze and cool temperatures were a relief from the heat of the day. There was a light fragrant scent carried on the breeze. The lambs were nestled together with their moms, leaning their heads on their moms' bodies. The moms' heads were inclined toward the babies. There, I felt a quiet joy—that all was well with the flock, with me, with the world. I felt *wholly safe*. My brain and nervous system were in a completely regulated state—and as a result I felt emotionally and physically safe.

Now think about the last time that you felt creative energy. It might have been during a writing project, a work of art, or a reorganization of your kitchen pantry. As you reflect on that situation, complete this sentence: *When I was working on X, I felt Y*. My sentence looks like this: When I was working on this book, I felt energized and expansive.

When we feel safe, our brain and nervous system are free to enjoy open, curious, creative exploration. In a regulated state, we can access the higher brain structures and functions so that we generate new ideas. When our brain and nervous system are dysregulated, the singular goal is survival, and the parts of our brain that become activated do so in service of making us safe.

Emotional Regulation

Emotional regulation is the ability to manage our emotions effectively—what we feel, when we feel, and how we express what we feel.[10] Someone with high emotional regulation doesn't allow their emotions to overtake their actions. Instead, they are thoughtful about how they express emotions.[11] The picture of emotional dys-regulation, when we can't put the brake on our negative emotions, looks like this:

- Negative thoughts and emotions dominate our daily experience.
- We feel like we're on a roller coaster of up-and-down emotions.
- We feel emotionally vulnerable or sensitive so that the slightest ill-timed or misplaced comment makes us feel hurt or angry.
- We feel frustrated, irritable, and angry, and we lash out as our emotions explode like a volcano.
- Our negative emotions spill out into our behaviour, so that we find ourselves in relationship conflict, behaving impulsively, using substances for relief.
- We experience symptoms of depression, anxiety, and stress.

Controlling our emotions is not the sole responsibility of our mind and will. We now understand that the gut-brain axis—the linkages between our gut, brain, nervous system, and hormonal and immune systems—play a central role in emotional regulation.[12] In fact, the gut is now referred to as the "second brain" because the brain and the gut are in constant communication. Caring for your brain and nervous system using the strategies in this book will have spillover effects of helping your gut to be healthy so that you may experience less gastrointestinal upset. And recent research shows that the health of a mother's gut-brain axis affects the development of the baby's gut-brain axis.[13]

Research from the ACEs studies show that when our nervous system is dysregulated, our ability to regulate our emotions is reduced, so that we are emotionally reactive, unable to modulate emotional responses, and inappropriate in our reactions.[14, 15] But we have the capacity to exercise choice around our emotions when our brain and nervous system are emotionally regulated, and it begins with identifying when our emotions are heightened and taking steps to manage them (a top-down strategy). A 2020 review of several research studies showed that this reflection, or reappraisal, is associated with well-being, as is our ability to accept the situation.[16]

Jack Canfield and Stephen Covey have shared a tool using this principle, which we have found helpful in our work: E + R = O, where E is the event or situation, R is your response, and O is the outcome. Your response (your thoughts, words, actions, and emotions) is what stands between the situation you face and the outcome. You may not be able to control the event, but you can control your response, and that's what determines how that situation turns out.[17, 18]

The wisdom of "Take a deep breath and count to ten when you're upset" is built on this principle. It works! Counting to ten when faced with a difficult experience gives time to pause and make a conscious choice about a response. Neurologically, the deep breath applies pressure to your vagal nerve, which sends a signal to your brain that says, "It's all okay. Everything is fine. I am calm and safe."

Self-acceptance

Self-acceptance is the ability to accept your whole self—both strengths and limitations. The opposite—not accepting ourselves—manifests when we beat ourselves up, criticize ourselves for not doing something differently or better, experience self-loathing, replay and scrutinize our words and actions, and believe that what we do is never enough. We carry around disappointment with ourselves, and fear and tension that others are disappointed with us. The problem is that self-acceptance tends to be hinged to an embedded belief system about how we view ourselves and our relationships with others. We experience a lack of safety, believing that we aren't "good enough" and that others see us that way as well. And it keeps us on high alert, hypervigilant to others' responses to us.

Not accepting ourselves keeps our nervous system in a chronically dysregulated state. One bottom-up strategy that can restore a sense of safety and regulation is Linda Graham's Hand on Heart exercise: put your right hand over your heart; take deep breaths to activate your body's calming, parasympathetic system; and think about a time when you were with someone who made you feel safe. This simple exercise helps your oxytocin to flow, which is a "feel-good" hormone that your body releases when it senses safety and security.[19]

Trusting Relationships, Social Connectedness, and Protectiveness

We are biologically and emotionally wired for social connection. Soothing experiences in utero and after birth, and positive parenting that uses gentle touch and responsive care are the bases of attachment that program our nervous system so that we can have trusting, satisfying, reciprocal relationships.[20, 21] In the consistent absence of these building blocks, the trajectory of brain and nervous system development is interrupted, stress hormones are elevated, and brain fear circuits are activated.[22, 23] Without a strong sense of connection, attachment, and belonging built on trust and empathy, our brain and nervous system become dysregulated and our risk for poor mental health in adulthood increases.[24] In his book *The Body Keeps the Score*, Dr. Bessel van der Kolk notes, "Being able to feel safe with other people is probably the single most important aspect of mental health; safe connections are fundamental to meaningful and satisfying lives."[25]

According to author and psychologist Dr. Henry Cloud, positive relationships are those where the other person wants the best for you.[26] They accept you just as you are without judgment, invite you to show your weaknesses and downsides, love you no matter who you are or what you do, help you to love better, cheer you on, energize you, give you honest feedback, respect your boundaries and autonomy, and help you to thrive and grow as a person. On the other hand, unsafe people tend to be controlling, judgmental, domineering, defensive, dishonest, and destructive.

There are other kinds of relationships that aren't unsafe per se, but they're not good connections. In these relationships, the interactions aren't positive or meaningful, but rather shallow and disengaging. These include what Dr. Cloud calls fake relationships: those that enamor you and make you feel good in the moment but ultimately leave you dissatisfied.[27]

We first learn how to regulate our nervous system as infants in the presence of a tender caregiver. We are closest to others when we feel understood and appreciated, engage in meaningful talk, do fun things together, and don't feel self-conscious. We don't have to put up walls to protect ourselves—there is a natural openness. Within the context of such relationships, we feel safe, and our nervous system is regulated. As adults, we benefit from co-regulation when we form a trusting, safe relationship that physiologically regulates the nervous system of both parties. When you nurture your brain health through safe relationships, you help your unborn child to experience the safety that is so critical for their brain development.

Safe connections always involve exercising boundaries. They are a necessary and normal part of every relationship we have—and our truly safe relationships make this easy for us. When I think of boundaries, I can't help but think of our sheep farm. When we first bought the farm, we spent one full year planning and designing the fencing system before we ever pounded our first post into the ground. We knew the importance of the fences in keeping our sheep in, keeping predators out, and in defining the land we care for versus what our neighbour manages. And fence checking and maintenance is a part of our daily work. We vigilantly walk the fences, making sure that they are intact so that our sheep remain safe.

Personal boundaries are just like our sheep fences. They provide a clear delineation of who is me, what is mine, and what I am about. They keep us safe from untoward influences. They help us to know what is ours to manage and what is not. And diligently maintaining and checking our personal boundaries is no less critical than walking the fences on our farm.

There are excellent resources on how to set and maintain boundaries. The two very best resources that I have personally used and recommend to my clients are Dr. Henry Cloud's *Boundaries*[28] and Nedra Glover Tawwab's *The Set Boundaries Workbook*.[29] These resources will literally change your life and relationships by helping you uncover the reasons you don't set or find it hard to set boundaries, and then showing you how to set boundaries that you can hold without feeling guilt or shame.

Sense of Safety

One of the key foundations of neuroscience is that the brain and nervous system are regulated when they sense safety, and dysregulated when they detect inescapable danger.[30] This isn't a new concept—we've known it for decades. But we are only starting to recognize that mental health relies upon supporting the brain and nervous system to achieve a sense of safety, from which regulation will flow.[31]

Dr. Stephen Porges describes levels of neurological activation that we experience with decreasing degrees of safety. When our brain first detects a threat in our environment, our brain and nervous system automatically initiate the first guard of attack—seek social connection. We call out for help and aid from those around us. When no one responds to our cry for help, our nervous system readies all our bodily systems necessary to stand and fight or run and escape. When we can't escape because we are (or feel) trapped and immobilized, then our nervous system moves into a freeze state where we collapse physically and emotionally, hoping that the attacker won't notice us and will leave. We don't speak or move, we conserve our energy, and we physically try to make our body smaller (e.g., by slouching, going into fetal position). Fawning is a stage we enter when all else has failed and the only relief we can hope for from the terrifyingly unsafe situation we are in is to try to please and cooperate with our attacker.

A first step to improving your sense of safety is to recognize the signals your body gives you when you feel unsafe, then re-regulating your nervous system through the Safe and Sound Protocol (see Chapter 7). Even if your system has been dysregulated your whole life, it can be re-regulated with these tools.

Healthy Coping Skills

Coping skills are anything we consciously or subconsciously do to reduce distress. Healthy coping skills help us to feel better and strengthen our ability to get through a difficult time so that we grow as a result. Negative ones help us to feel somewhat better but tend to keep us stuck in the situation and often come with negative consequences; for example, suppressing grief may help us to feel better in the moment but leaves the pain unresolved so that it continues to wear on us.

Healthy coping skills have always been thought of as top-down strategies that we intentionally use for managing life's challenges and building resilience. But sometimes our brain and nervous system are so dysregulated we can't put top-down coping skills into action. By combining them with bottom-up strategies to regulate and maintain regulation of our brain and nervous system, we can maximize the effectiveness of healthy coping skills and ensure our mental health flourishes.

Here are some coping strategies that reduce clinical symptoms of depression, anxiety, and stress and improve mental health:

- Social activities: spending time with family and friends
- Personal recreation, hobbies, or interests
- Pursuing goals: working on something that gives you a sense of achievement and fulfills your need for purpose
- Spiritual practices such as praying and meditating

These strategies are effective primarily because they have a regulatory effect on our nervous system. Building *safe* social connections talking to a friend, sitting with other people even in shared stillness, sending a text to a friend, and imagining being with a friend—is the most healthful thing we can do for our nervous system.[32] Personal recreation and hobbies, especially those done in connection with others, capitalize on the value of play, which also has a toning effect on the nervous system, especially when they don't involve screens.[33] Pursuing goals helps us to exercise those parts of our brain that are designed to create and which are locked down when we are in a dysregulated state. Finally, research has shown that spiritual practices improve brain structure and function through enhanced neuroplasticity.[34]

In *The Polyvagal Theory in Therapy*, Deb Dana writes about the principle of matching our regulatory strategies to the state of our nervous system. When we are highly dysregulated in a "freeze" state where we are immobilized and shut down, we need the co-regulation of a trusted person to help us to re-regulate our nervous system. In this case, a visit with a friend is the best strategy. When we are slightly dysregulated in a fight-or-flight state, running on the treadmill will allow our nervous energy to dissipate and our nervous system to regulate. When we are regulated, playing sports, or making art help us to stay in the higher centres of our brain. Our choice of coping skill or regulatory strategy is most effective when we intentionally match it to the state of our nervous system.

Sense of Purpose

A person who is flourishing emotionally (and physically) has a strong sense of meaning and purpose that guides their life decisions, allows them to achieve meaningful goals, and helps them contribute to the lives of others in significant ways. Not only do they tend to live longer but they also have less cognitive decline as they age, half the chance of aging with Alzheimer's disease, and fewer age-related brain changes.

A sense of purpose is one of the most important markers of mental health because it acts as a North Star when we experience setbacks and adversity. It bubbles out above life's challenges, helping us to discern the story of what difficult experiences mean to us and how they relate to our calling and significance on this earth. Holocaust survivor Viktor Frankl is a model of someone who understood the value of purpose in moving through great adversity. Regarding his fellow inmates, he noted, "Whenever there was an opportunity for it, one had to give them a why—an aim—for their lives, in order to strengthen them to bear the terrible how of their existence. Woe to him who saw no more sense in his life, no aim, no purpose, and therefore no point in carrying on. He was soon lost."[35]

In his book *The Second Mountain*, David Brooks describes how many people's lives follow a two-mountain structure.[36] He says of people on the first mountain: "They get out of school, they start a career, and they begin climbing the mountain they thought they were meant to climb. Their goals on this first mountain are the ones our culture endorses: to be a success, to make your mark, to experience personal happiness. But when they get to the top of that mountain, something happens. They look around and find the view . . . unsatisfying. They realize: This wasn't my mountain after all. There's another, bigger mountain out there that's actually my mountain." Can you relate? I can!

Brooks goes on to describe the second mountain, one that espouses a life of meaning and purpose. He notes that the second mountain may arise out of adversity and suffering and may involve radical life changes or dramatic attitudinal shifts. Those journeying on their second mountain do so girded with the elements that make them a whole person.

In my counselling work, I find that many women embark upon a second mountain of sorts during pregnancy. They begin to raise questions about the role of their career in their lives or the way they've operated in their career pre-pregnancy. Some begin a second mountain with a determination to disrupt certain intergenerational patterns. They begin the journey of moving beyond others' expectations to fulfill their own purpose.

Many books and online resources are available to help people find a greater sense of their life's purpose, but you can start small by giving some thought to this statement that was designed by a friend and colleague, Dr. Michael Frisina: *My purpose in life is to express my core values of X through my love of Y and my unique talents of Z.*

Growth Mindset

How we feel about our ability to learn and grow is also important to our mental health. Stanford University researcher Carol Dweck became interested over thirty years ago in students' attitudes toward failure and success at school. Out of that work, she described the growth mindset as the belief that we can change, develop our abilities, and overcome difficulties. She and her team found that not only was a growth mindset associated with good mental health but also that people with a growth mindset embraced learning as a process, feedback for improvement, and mistakes as learning opportunities.[37, 38, 39] As a result, they set and achieved their goals. They also benefitted from experience-dependent neuroplasticity because as they allowed themselves to learn from life experiences, their brains were stimulated to reorganize their neuronal networks, resulting in a healthier brain.

On the other end of the spectrum were those who held a fixed mindset. They were mired in the belief that their abilities were capped at birth and that their intelligence and skills were therefore limited by their genetics. They tended to take feedback personally, interpreted making mistakes as personal failure, avoided making mistakes, and gave up easily or didn't try. It wasn't that they were willful, lazy, or unmotivated—words that perhaps you remember from your childhood. It was that they were immobilized and inhibited by their belief that they would never rise above their genetics or their abilities at that point in time and would always be relegated to second best or failure.

Take a moment to reflect on which mindset you have, but let me first outline three key ideas that will help you to have perspective and self-compassion.

First, we know a lot more about neuroplasticity than we did thirty years ago when work on growth mindset began, and this new science gives cause for much hope. From a neurobiological perspective, our brains are capable of change (and healing) *throughout our lives*. The idea that we can't change or learn beyond childhood and adolescence is just old science that lives on as myth.

Second, early childhood experiences shape our mindset. For instance, a child who was criticized for poor marks may believe that they lack intelligence and avoid educational pursuits as an adult. Another who had to work hard at school subjects might interpret their efforts as "I'm dumb" and not go on to achieve what they love and are best at. Have self-compassion around your fixed mindset because it is likely that it came at a high personal cost of pain, discouragement, and hardship.

Third, it isn't uncommon to have a growth mindset in one area (for example, our job) and a fixed mindset in another (perhaps the belief that our parents weren't nurturing and we're destined to be the same).

Research also shows that parents' mindset around failure influences their parenting and their responses to their children's failure, which in turn affects their children's mindsets.[40] For instance, parents who hold the mindset that failure is debilitating tend to have children with fixed mindsets, while those with the mindset that failure is enhancing have children with growth mindsets. It is worth considering our own mindset so that we can grow our own mental health and intentionally foster the growth we desire for our children. Remember: your brain is neuroplastic, capable of creating new neural pathways that foster new beliefs and thoughts.

To build a growth mindset, exercise self-compassion as a priority. Take the word *fail* out of your vocabulary and replace it with *learn*. Language is an important aid to helping you to restructure your beliefs. Another strategy is to view challenges and difficulties as opportunities to grow and stretch.

Autonomy

Humans have a psychological need for autonomy; that is, we need to feel that we have choice and the power to exercise it. Although we are built for connection with others, we are also emotionally and cognitively designed to be separate from others. In fact, good parenting helps children to transition comfortably and safely from co-dependence to dependence. I have served women in my counselling practice who have been shaped by enmeshed families where being a good person and family member hinge on wide-open sharing— and agreement—on all life decisions. The resulting guilt, shame, and anxiety, not to mention relationship dysfunction (for example, threat of expulsion from the family), is unbearable.

Autonomy doesn't mean that we don't need or rely on other people. It means that we have a good balance between independence and dependence so that we can make our own decisions and set healthy boundaries *and* experience connection with others. It means being aware of and comfortable with our own likes and dislikes, wishes, needs, and opinions while showing equal respect for others in these areas.

Ultimately, autonomy is an expression of our safety in relationships and, therefore, a reflection of our brain and nervous system's level of regulation. As Deb Dana notes, "Free to share, to stay, to leave . . ." characterizes a safe relationship where both individuals have autonomy. [41] A person who is dysregulated may not feel that they can make their own decisions, may believe they don't have permission to have and express needs and opinions, and may not feel they have the right to set boundaries. They don't have a sense of self that says, "I am me, and you are you."

We're not born with a lack of autonomy, but it happens when we've not been encouraged or allowed to express our personal needs, values, and opinions. This can occur if we've been given a message that our opinions weren't important, or if we've experienced negative consequences when we have expressed them, such as emotional blackmail or withdrawal. I can't tell you how many women (and men!) I counselled who were not given permission to express their needs or wants, and who look at me blankly when I ask, "What do you need?" These early experiences rewire our nervous system so that relationships become a source of threat instead of safety. Speaking out our opinion or needs places us in a vulnerable position of being rejected, hurt, or harmed. In other words, when we lack autonomy, we inherently feel unsafe to give our own opinion, express our needs, make decision, or set boundaries.

How do you increase your autonomy?

1. Set boundaries around people who are unsafe in your life. Another of Dr. Henry Cloud's books, *Safe People*, is an excellent resource that will help you identify who is unsafe in your life (we might be so caught in the relationship pattern that we are unable to recognize who is unsafe and the effects on us) and how to set and maintain boundaries that protect you from them. [42]

2. Know your values, likes, dislikes, and opinions. For some, it will seem that the last sentence was written in a foreign

language. You've never sensed that you've had permission to express yourself in this manner. If this is you, start by completing this sentence: *I am at my best when I . . .* Make a list of all the things that help you to be at your best. These are your needs and likes!

3. In a safe, trusted relationship, start to articulate what's important to you. Then, practice. Think of it as your personal research project, with no pressure of how things turn out. Experiment with and study the outcomes of what happens when you speak your values, opinions, needs, likes, and wants. Listen carefully, then introduce your thoughts with statements such as, "That's interesting. For me, . . ." or, "I believe . . ." or, "In my experience . . ." or, "My impression is that . . ." Learn to express yourself with calm, composed authenticity. If you don't have a safe personal relationship, a counsellor can play this role for you.

Psychological Flexibility

Another sign of mental health is psychological flexibility—being able to accept life's realities and adapt to its demands. For a moment, think of a time when you consciously accepted an unexpected circumstance. Can you feel yourself relax and breathe deeply? You've moved past the fact that it happened, and you are open and ready to mobilize resources for moving forward. In a recent study of more than 400 adolescents, all of whom had experienced adverse childhood experiences (ACEs), psychological flexibility was the only difference between those who developed depression symptoms and those who did not.[43] In a follow-up commentary to this landmark article, another researcher identified psychological flexibility as "the ACE we need."[44]

The opposite, resistance, is when we refuse to accept our circumstances. We don't generally blatantly stand on our balcony and shout, "I refuse to accept that this happened to me!" No, it's much more subtle than that. Resistance is an inner state filled with tension and conflict because rather than accepting and moving forward in the situation, we expend energy and emotion being stuck at the beginning, in angst that the situation happened to us in the first place. Recent research in a group of adults who had experienced childhood adversity showed that the tendency to ruminate about their past interfered with their ability to accept and move forward, so that their lives were characterized by "constantly thinking about the past," "not being able to move away from childhood traumas," "not being able to forgive their parents," "inability to get rid of negative thoughts," "living in the past," and "suppression of emotions."[45] Perhaps you can relate. They lived their lives locked up (suppressed), like a volcano that continued to build heat and fury with no release.

I've personally experienced resistance and the angst that it entailed. While writing this book, my mother passed away. Although she had been ill for some time, her death was still unexpected, and I found it difficult to accept that I was living in a world without my mother. I would often say inwardly and outwardly, "I don't want it to be this way! I don't want to be in the Daughters Without Mothers Club." During grief counselling, I discovered the work of Dr. Alan Wolfelt, who described the process of reconciliation as "the serenity to become comfortable with the way things are rather than attempting to make things as they were." I loved that. I felt peaceful just reading it.

In subsequent grief and loss research, I learned that a key part of accepting a blindsiding experience in our lives is to "rewrite" our journey. Someone who is flourishing has the flexibility to shift their mindset, perspective, and behaviour in response to a challenging life circumstance. That doesn't mean that they are happy that a difficult situation has arisen in their life—who is? It means that their nervous system is regulated sufficiently so they can experience—and recover from—hardship. They don't stagnate and ruminate over the fact that a difficult thing has happened. They're psychologically flexible, and that builds resilience.

When I think about what it's like to ruminate, I picture our sheep. Sheep are ruminant animals, which means that after they have finished grazing grass or eating hay, they ruminate. They stand or lay down in the pasture, close their eyes to narrow slits, regurgitate bits of what they have swallowed, and re-chew their cud—over and over again. They'll chew for several minutes in a rhythmic, side-to-side chewing pattern. It's an automatic part of normal digestion for them. It's healthy for them, but not for us! When we ruminate about a situation, we replay it repeatedly, over and over again—just like the sheep and their cud. We hold it in our mind. We think about it, worry about it, and let our fears run amuck over it. It's like watching the same movie scene, repeatedly pushing the "back 30 seconds" button.

From a brain perspective, rumination is unhealthy because it strengthens those brain neural circuits involved in the repetitive, negative thoughts—making it easier and more automatic to have unhealthy thought patterns. Picture your brain as a multi-laned highway with several overpasses crisscrossing overhead. When you repeatedly think a negative thought, that thought travels along the same brain highway, over and over, creating a well-entrenched path for other negative thoughts to follow. When you think a new thought, your brain's electrical impulses redirect and travel along a new brain circuit. The more you use that new, healthy highway the easier it becomes for subsequent healthy thoughts to flow down that path.

The effects of rumination and inflexibility aren't just limited to our brain. If they were, they'd only affect us. When we are psychologically inflexible, not accepting life's circumstances, we tend to be irritable, angry, frustrated, depressed, and anxious.[46] These reactions seep into our personal and professional relationships, creating tension, conflict, and angst. For this reason, many clinicians and researchers highlight psychological flexibility as one of the most important aspects of mental health. The more flexible you are, the more likely you are to accept and adjust to changes in your life circumstances, and the easier it is for you to bounce back or be resilient.

Are you wondering just how psychologically flexible you are? The following assessment is a series of ten questions that can help you assess your psychological flexibility.

SELF-ASSESSMENT

The Psychological Flexibility Scale

Below is a list of twelve experiences. Using the scale (Never true to Always true), indicate how often you experienced the situation in each statement over the past two weeks. Then, sum up the totals for statements 1 through 6 to find your flexibility score and the totals for statements 7 through 12 to find your inflexibility score.

In the last two weeks . . .

1. I tried to make peace with my negative thoughts and feelings rather than resisting them.

Never true	Rarely true	Occasionally true	Often true	Very often true	Always true
1	2	3	4	5	6

2. I paid close attention to what I was thinking and feeling.

Never true	Rarely true	Occasionally true	Often true	Very often true	Always true
1	2	3	4	5	6

3. Even when I felt hurt or upset, I tried to maintain a broader perspective.

Never true	Rarely true	Occasionally true	Often true	Very often true	Always true
1	2	3	4	5	6

4. In tough situations, I was able to notice my thoughts and feelings without getting overwhelmed by them.

Never true	Rarely true	Occasionally true	Often true	Very often true	Always true
1	2	3	4	5	6

5. I was very in touch with what is important to me and my life.

Never true	Rarely true	Occasionally true	Often true	Very often true	Always true
1	2	3	4	5	6

6. Even when I stumbled in my efforts, I didn't quit working toward what is important.

Never true	Rarely true	Occasionally true	Often true	Very often true	Always true
1	2	3	4	5	6

Your flexibility score (sum of statements 1 to 6):

7. When something unpleasant came up, I tried very hard to stop thinking about it.

Never true	Rarely true	Occasionally true	Often true	Very often true	Always true
1	2	3	4	5	6

8. I did most things on "auto-pilot" with little awareness of what I was doing.

Never true	Rarely true	Occasionally true	Often true	Very often true	Always true
1	2	3	4	5	6

9. I thought some of my emotions were bad or inappropriate and I shouldn't feel them.

Never true	Rarely true	Occasionally true	Often true	Very often true	Always true
1	2	3	4	5	6

10. Negative thoughts and feelings tended to stick with me for a long time.

Never true	Rarely true	Occasionally true	Often true	Very often true	Always true
1	2	3	4	5	6

11. When life got hectic, I often lost touch with the things I value.

Never true	Rarely true	Occasionally true	Often true	Very often true	Always true
1	2	3	4	5	6

12. Negative feelings often trapped me in inaction.

Never true	Rarely true	Occasionally true	Often true	Very often true	Always true
1	2	3	4	5	6

Your inflexibility score (sum of statements 7 to 12):

Your Results

Your results comprise two scores: a flexibility score and an inflexibility score. The higher your *flexibility* score, the better your ability to adapt to change. As a rule of thumb, a score of 30 to 36 indicates high flexibility, 20 to 29 is moderate, and less than 20 is low.

The psychological inflexibility score (the total of questions 7 to 12) ranges from the lowest score of 6 to a highest score of 36. The higher your *inflexibility* score, the more likely you are to struggle with change. A score of 30 to 36 indicates high inflexibility, 20 to 29 is moderate inflexibility, and less than 20 is low psychological inflexibility, indicating that you generally accept and readily adjust to change in your approaches or situation.[47]

As you reflect on your results, remember that psychological inflexibility, like a fever, can be a sign of some underlying neurological dysregulation. There is no room for shame or guilt. Psychological inflexibility is most often the result of childhood adversity that has rewired your brain to see safety in sameness and threat in change. As I say to my clients, "It would be normal for the abnormal experience you had."

Other strategies that are effective for increasing your psychological flexibility are knowing what your values are. People who struggle with psychological inflexibility, especially around past adversities, don't live a value-driven life. They are consumed by the past rather than living out their values—what's important to them—in the present.[48] There are several lists of values online that ask you to simply read the list and circle those that resonate with you. Or you can make a list of answers in response to the statement: *It is important to me that . . .* For example, what comes up for me is: *It is important to me that I am kind and compassionate to others.* Being explicit about your values by putting words to them will allow you to adjust your perspective and thinking to be in line with what's important to you. Then, when you need to make a change, you can do it in a way that maintains the essence of what is important to you.

Another strategy is to recognize and appreciate your patterns of thoughts and feelings of being stuck or immobilized. Part of the problem of being psychologically inflexible is that it's often unconscious. We resist moving forward because we're confused, afraid, protecting ourselves, or trying desperately to get us back to a place where we were once safe and secure and happy. Being stuck is often accompanied by feeling restricted, confined, frustrated, sad, and/or stressed—the painful opposite of an open mind.

Recognize those emotions for what they are—signals that you are digging your heels in—by asking yourself this series of questions: What is keeping me in this place? What had I hoped for? What absolute truths am I hanging on to? What rigid beliefs about the way things must be are keeping me stuck in this place? What is my greatest worry or fear in moving forward? What are the costs to moving forward? What are the benefits? What is made possible by moving beyond this place? By answering these questions, you'll gain some personal insight about how inflexibility is affecting your life and begin to open up to new directions and possibilities.

Sense of Control

Feeling that we are in control and able to manage our lives is another important part of mental health. Someone who is flourishing feels that they are in control of their life and believes that they have what is needed to manage their relationships, parenting, and career. They create and execute goals and have a positive view of the future. When there is ambiguity in their lives, they put in place certain structures, decisions, and boundaries to regain their sense of control. If their situation can't change, they adjust their emotions and thoughts.

Someone who lacks a sense of control may feel that they don't have the ability to set goals or plan their future. They may lose interest and feel hopeless about their future or experience overwhelm, frustration, anger, stress, and anxiety. Our brain needs to feel that it has control—especially to escape danger—to feel safe. The most impactful traumatic events are those where our brain has interpreted the situation as inescapable.

If you have a deep sense that you don't have control in your life, that things happen to you, and you are powerless to respond, try setting goals and taking steps to accomplish them. Over time, your sense of control will naturally grow as you gain confidence in your ability to meet goals. That will give you even greater confidence to set other more challenging goals.

Cultivation of Positive Emotions

Negative and positive emotions have very different effects on our brains and bodies. Negative emotions engage our sympathetic nervous system, launching us into fight-or-flight mode. Our attention narrows as we become laser-focused on the threat, our metabolic and cardiac systems are aroused to increase our heart rate, breathing, and blood pressure, and our non-essential functions (when you're fighting for your life), such as digestion, slow down.

Conversely, positive emotions activate the parasympathetic branch of our nervous system, which reduces our metabolism, muscle tension, and blood pressure, slows our heart rate and breathing, and makes us feel at rest and at peace. Instead of narrowing our thinking, we become expansive, creative, and flexible.

While our emotions affect our brain and body, there is a bidirectional relationship where our brain and nervous system also signal our emotions. Think about the last time you were driving and saw a vehicle coming toward you out of the corner of your eye. Long before you registered the potential accident in the thinking parts of your brain, your inner lighthouse (e.g., your amygdala) detected the threat. You *felt* fear before your brain *registered* fear in the form of a thought. While these are the actions of a healthy nervous system— alerting us to danger when danger exists—a dysregulated nervous system tends to flood us with negative emotions regularly—or constantly. We feel under threat, worried, anxious, stressed, and fearful.

Top-down strategies (e.g., change your thinking so that your emotions will change) include shifting your emotions. Many women have used suppression—stuffing their emotions down—as a coping mechanism, and it has served them well.[49] For short periods of time, it can be useful. A few years ago, I underwent chemotherapy for stage II breast cancer. Every two weeks for four months

I spent my Saturday morning in the infusion room at our regional cancer centre receiving chemotherapy. For those four months, I didn't allow myself to process the cancer diagnosis or the treatment. I suppressed my emotions and just did what I had to do. Then, a few months after the chemotherapy was finished, I processed it all—the diagnosis, the treatment, and how I felt about it all. I didn't know I was in suppression—it wasn't something I one day decided to do. It was subconscious. I felt that if I allowed myself to feel pain around the diagnosis and treatment, I would sink into a large hole that I would not climb out of easily. I couldn't verbalize this at the time, but in hindsight I could see that it was the unspoken fear. I simply did what I needed to do—and then I processed it all. Perhaps you can relate.

However, research is clear that when we chronically suppress our emotions, we are at risk for depression, anxiety, eating disorders, and substance use.[50] Long term, it's just not healthy. That's why I recommend that you start with a bottom-up approach to regulate your nervous system as this will give you the capacity to effectively use top-down strategies. The easiest place to start is five minutes of deep breathing, because it requires very little of us except to take a deep breath in through the nose, allowing your belly to expand, for a count of four and slowly exhale for a count of six.

The Positive and Negative Affect (Emotion) Schedule is an assessment tool that can help you know whether your emotions tend toward positivity or negativity. It was first published more than thirty years ago and has been used clinically and in research studies to help draw connections between emotional states and health outcomes.

The Positive and Negative Affect Schedule[51]

The goal of this assessment is to help you reflect on the balance of positive and negative emotions you've experienced the past two weeks. Simply indicate how many times you've felt the given emotion, then tally emotions 1 through 10 for your positive emotion score and tally emotions 11 through 20 for your negative emotion score.

EMOTION	Very slightly or not at all	A little	Moderately	Quite a bit	Extremely
1. Active	1	2	3	4	5
2. Alert	1	2	3	4	5
3. Attentive	1	2	3	4	5
4. Determined	1	2	3	4	5
5. Enthusiastic	1	2	3	4	5
6. Excited	1	2	3	4	5
7. Inspired	1	2	3	4	5
8. Interested	1	2	3	4	5
9. Proud	1	2	3	4	5
10. Strong	1	2	3	4	5

Your total positive emotion score of questions 1 through 10:

EMOTION	Very slightly or not at all	A little	Moderately	Quite a bit	Extremely
11. Afraid	1	2	3	4	5
12. Scared	1	2	3	4	5
13. Nervous	1	2	3	4	5
14. Jittery	1	2	3	4	5
15. Irritable	1	2	3	4	5
16. Hostile	1	2	3	4	5
17. Guilty	1	2	3	4	5
18. Ashamed	1	2	3	4	5
19. Upset	1	2	3	4	5
20. Distressed	1	2	3	4	5
Your total negative emotion score of questions 11 through 20:					

Your Results

Your results are composed of two scores: your positive emotion score and your negative emotion score. The higher your score in either category, the higher your level of those emotions over the last two weeks. Remember that it's all about balance. Negative emotions are a normal part of life, and some days we experience more than others. We have better emotional health when we don't ignore or suppress them, and instead learn to acknowledge, tolerate, and manage them. It's when we experience strong, negative emotions for a prolonged period that the balance of our emotional health tips to the *unhealthy* side.

If you experience negative emotions most days, and they are interfering with your life and relationships, reflect on whether they might have originated from a single experience or an accumulation of life challenges or trauma—in childhood or adulthood. If so, your nervous system is likely dysregulated and you should look to cultivate positive emotions, which is just as important as dialing down—or deregulating—negative ones. Here are several research-based strategies to upregulating positive emotions:

- Allow yourself to laugh
- Create positive sensory events, such as beautiful sights, scents, music, tactile objects that feel good (e.g., soft blanket), massages, and warm baths
- Nurture gratitude (e.g., regularly reflect on/write about things you are grateful for)
- Create goals and plans to meet them, especially around activities that you find life-giving
- Perform guided imagery (using muscle relaxation and positive mental images to produce psychological and physiological relaxation)
- Share or write about positive experiences
- Foster connections with significant friends and family
- Exercise
- Immerse yourself in nature

As a bonus, research shows that when you up-regulate your positive emotions, the benefits are far-reaching, including greater happiness, life satisfaction, and self-esteem.

Good Mental Health During Pregnancy

I've been discussing what comprises mental health in general, and I'd like to focus now on how to foster mental health in the midst of a significant transition, such as pregnancy. Change is, by its very nature, off-balancing. I think the word roots for *change* put a particularly interesting spin on our common understanding: to exchange, bend, become crooked/curved, substitute something for something else. I love that because it speaks to the personal shifts that are inevitable during transition. We change!

How we approach change dictates whether we walk through transition in a regulated, healthy way or a chaotic, unregulated state. In his excellent book *Necessary Endings*, Dr. Henry Cloud notes, "If a situation falls within the range of normal, expected, and known, the human brain automatically marshals all available resources and moves to engage it. But if the brain interprets the situation as negative, dangerous, wrong, or unknown, a fight-or-flight response kicks in that moves us *away* from the issue or begins to resist it."[52] Pregnancies that are high risk can certainly propel women into a state of sympathetic nervous activation as they face constant uncertainty about their own and their baby's health. But many women with low-risk pregnancies still find the unknown—the uncertainty— around the pregnancy, labour, and delivery trying.

To walk a new path in a neurobiologically healthy way means accepting and adjusting to a new reality like pregnancy, your changing role and identity, and your shifting family life. The key pillars of managing transition well involve:

- Knowing yourself—your core values, beliefs, personality, likes/dislikes, and triggers—and living according to your values, convictions, priorities, and boundaries, even though you're navigating new waters.
- Managing your emotions so that you accept and acknowledge negative emotions that may arise as you face change and trials, but move readily back into a positive state, protecting your inner well-being and outer relationships.
- Accepting your whole self—including the great parts and the "areas under construction"—and having self-compassion when the sand is shifting under your feet.
- Trusting a significant other who is worthy of your trust so that you have someone to walk with along your new path.
- Coping by moving through the transition or difficulty headstrong, like a ship plowing across the ocean swells, rather than retreating and avoiding, and growing, personally and interpersonally.
- Building your story of this season of transition (What does this change mean to you? For some, pregnancy is the end of a long and stress-filled infertility journey).
- Growing—in yourself and your relationships—although the change or hard times challenge the very fibre of your being.
- Possessing the inner confidence and outer competence that will help you to walk along your new path.

Change of any variety can be especially difficult for some women. Depending on our early life experiences, some of us are wired to interpret change as dangerous and threatening. We simply cannot embrace change as positive. We can't even begin to put those pillars of healthy change into place. If this resonates with you, turn to Chapter 7 and begin to put the BEE Protocol into place. This will help you immensely, not only in your pregnancy, but across all areas of your life.

As we've walked through what it means to have good mental health, the bottom line is this: Good mental health begins—and ends—with a regulated brain and nervous system. New neuroscience has taught us how to help the brain heal itself so that no matter what your starting point (depression, anxiety, stress, trauma), your brain and nervous system can be healthy.

Don't leave your mental health to chance.

CHAPTER 3

The Truth About Depression

"I had no idea. I wish I'd known earlier . . ."

This is the most common response I hear when, in my work as a counsellor, I tell new mothers with postpartum depression that their symptoms may have started *during* their pregnancy. And it's easy to understand why. When we think of depression and pregnancy, our minds instantly go to *postpartum* depression. This wasn't always the case. Mood swings, like depression in new mothers, were considered an exaggerated hormonal response to pregnancy and birth. But in 1994, our whole view of and approach to postpartum depression changed when it was officially classed as a psychiatric disorder in the fourth edition of the *Diagnostic and Statistical Manual of Mental Disorders* (DSM-IV), the medical bible of psychiatrists and psychologists. Prescription and usage of antidepressants in new mothers soared. Famous actresses shared their stories. News reports of postpartum psychosis and infanticides flooded the media.

We've had heightened awareness of depression in new mothers for over twenty years now. Some countries have responded with policies and practices that include mental health care as part of routine postpartum care. But, sadly, we have very little awareness of the significant numbers of women with prenatal depression, anxiety, and stress and little acknowledgement of the lifelong effects that babies carry as a result. And it isn't for lack of research! As you read in Chapter 1, we've known for over twenty-five years that the evidence is clear: mental health problems in pregnant women and animals cause deleterious, lifelong developmental consequences for babies.

It wasn't until 2013 that the committee that formulated the DSM-5 agreed to acknowledge that prenatal depression was a definable, real struggle for many pregnant women. But at the writing of this book, a decade later, we still lack routine prenatal mental health screening and care in most countries of the world. It is as if our maternal-child advocacy efforts stopped half-way, focusing on new mothers with babies and completely missing pregnant women with a vulnerable, growing fetus. In my view, the lack of response to the growing body of evidence clearly connecting poor mental health (aka nervous system dysregulation) in pregnancy with health and developmental challenges in the infant is intolerable and inexcusable.

The fact is that for 50 percent of women with PPD, the symptoms often begin *during* pregnancy, but many women—and doctors, for that matter—aren't on the lookout for signs of depression *before* birth, only *after*. And yet, over the past decade, research study after research study has shown that prenatal depression is just as common as postpartum depression. At 1 in 5 women experiencing symptoms of prenatal depression, a prenatal class of twenty women would have four that are struggling with depression. Compare that with some of the physical complications that doctors check for. Gestational diabetes occurs in 2 percent to 10 percent of pregnant women. High blood pressure develops in 5 percent to 8 percent.

Prenatal depression affects more women than either of these two conditions, but it generally goes undiagnosed.

This chapter will explain why that is and why it's important to watch for signs of depression earlier. I'll also explain the symptoms and warning signs—what emotions and feelings are normal and to be expected during pregnancy, and what are not. I'll discuss the causes and triggers of depression, so you have the information and tools to assess and safeguard your mental health. If you are concerned that you—or a loved one—may be experiencing depression during their pregnancy, know that you are not alone and help is within your grasp.

What Is Depression and What Does It Look Like in Pregnancy?

Jill's Story

I walked in the front door, exhausted from the workday, and immediately went to lay down on the couch. My partner, Josiah, was in the kitchen, making spaghetti, my favorite meal, by the smell of it. The thought of eating it tonight, though, brought tears to my eyes. I rubbed the small, round bump on my stomach. I should be happy, I knew. This was our first pregnancy. Josiah and I were so excited when we found out we were expecting. The first trimester had been tough—I had an especially bad case of morning sickness that left me drained, and the winter days had been particularly dark and cold. Everyone said things would get better in the second trimester, that I'd have a burst of energy, but I was twenty weeks, the days were warmer and longer, and yet it was taking all my physical and mental energy to do anything beyond the bare minimum. And there was so much to do—painting the baby's room, assembling the crib, and finding local prenatal classes. I hadn't even gotten out my summer clothes yet or bought seeds for the garden I always planted.

I felt a heavy weight settle on my chest. *What was wrong with me?* I thought, wiping a tear from my cheek. I loved my baby, more than anything, but how could I be a mother if I couldn't bring myself to do the basics?

Josiah came over to me. "Dinner in five," he said, then stopped, seeing my tears. "Mood swing?"

"I feel like I've been feeling this way for months. I feel so hopeless." I began to sob.

He held me in his arms. "I'm worried about you. This sounds like more than a mood swing. Could you be . . ." He trailed off.

"Depressed?" I finished for him.

He nodded.

It was a word I'd thought of more and more in the last weeks. I'd heard of postpartum depression, but never about depression during pregnancy. The thought made me feel like a failure, and I'd been afraid to give voice to it, until now.

I took a deep breath. "I don't know, but I think we need to find out."

—Jill, 20 weeks

In general, the symptoms of depression during pregnancy look similar to depression outside of pregnancy except that prenatal depression is more often combined with anxiety. But as Jill's story shows, it can be difficult to pick up on the warning signs of depression—like persistent feelings of sadness—because expecting mothers often experience mood swings. But the main difference with mood swings is that they are more like bouts of teariness that appear out of nowhere and fade as suddenly as they come. They can feel intense at the time, but they leave no lingering sadness or worry, have no impact on sleep or eating habits, and cause no change in your day-to-day energy levels. And they are a completely normal part of pregnancy. Pregnant women can have many mood swings over a period of weeks, but in between they feel like their normal (pregnant!) selves.

Prenatal depression also involves feelings of sadness and worry, but the difference is that these emotions last for a few weeks or longer. While you may feel less sad and worried at certain times than others, a general sense of sadness persists, and you don't feel like your normal self. Pregnant women with symptoms of depression often describe themselves as having a profound sadness that they just can't shake. They feel as though they've lost their joy and zest for life; things that once brought them pleasure and laughter no longer bring them happiness and contentment. They know their lives are not what they want them to be—and they feel guilty for it. This guilt and low self-confidence can be as much a challenge as the symptoms themselves.

Symptoms of Depression

Beyond feelings of sadness, the main symptoms of depression are:[1]

1. lowering of mood most of the day, nearly every day
2. markedly diminished interest or pleasure in all, or almost all, activities most of the day, nearly every day

3. significant weight loss when not dieting or significant weight gain (beyond pregnancy requirements), or decrease or increase in appetite nearly every day

4. a slowing down of thought and a reduction of activity

5. fatigue or loss of energy nearly every day

6. feelings of worthlessness (low self-esteem, low self-confidence) or excessive guilt nearly every day

7. diminished ability to think or concentrate, or indecisiveness, nearly every day

8. recurrent thoughts of death or suicide

Depending on the number and level of symptoms experienced, depression can range from mild to severe. Although this may feel like labelling, knowing what category your symptoms fit into helps with knowing what steps to take.

Women with *mild* depression have two or three symptoms, with the most common being not looking forward to things with enjoyment and not being able to laugh and see the funny side of things (number 2) and blaming themselves unnecessarily (number 6). The symptoms of mild depression are distressing because we don't feel like ourselves, but most women find that they can continue with their daily life. Does this mean we don't need to do something about mild symptoms? No—all levels of depression, even sub-clinical levels, warrant care. It's not unlike having a fever. When you have a mild fever, you might take a day off work and rest more. The fever is the signal that all is not well with your body, that there is an infection somewhere, and extra care is needed. Mild depression is a sign of brain and body dysregulation at an early stage for which you can use effective strategies to heal.

Women with *moderate* depression have four or more of these symptoms. They usually cry, feel sad or miserable, and are so unhappy that it interferes with sleeping, which is not on the list, but is common in pregnancy and postpartum. With moderate depression, most women struggle with ordinary social and professional activities to a degree. Jill experienced moderate depression, having struggled with low energy that left her unable to do some of the things she loved, hopelessness about whether she'd ever feel better, guilt about not seeing the doctor earlier, and loss of confidence about whether she could meet her baby's needs. Her low energy and mood were making it harder for her to cope with her daily work and home responsibilities.

To be diagnosed with *severe* prenatal depression, a woman would experience at least five or more of the eight symptoms within the same two-week period and feel like these symptoms were causing her significant distress socially and at home and work. The good news is that this is a small number of cases; most pregnant women with depression experience mild or moderate symptoms.

One of the most widespread myths is that depression in pregnant women disappears when their hormones calm down. In other words, depression that begins in pregnancy is caused by hormones and self-resolves at the end of pregnancy, but that's not the case, especially in the absence of appropriate care. Research conducted in many different countries shows that a significant number of women who experience depression in pregnancy continue to experience depression after their baby is born. It is hard to get a single statistic on the exact number of women who experience *chronic* depression, but it falls somewhere between 15 percent and 20 percent.[2, 3]

You'll remember that one of the causes of depression is dysregulation of our brain and nervous system that results from challenging life experiences.[4] Much of this research draws a strong connection between the long-lasting effects of childhood adversity on chronic depression, which also interrupts our brain's ability to self-heal through neuroplasticity.[5, 6]

It isn't a random throw of the dice that determines who develops chronic depression. Women who are most vulnerable have not had good social support.[7] Our team's research agrees with this and adds a history of depression or anxiety.[8] Their pattern of depression is different, too. These women develop *severe* symptoms in the first trimester, and their symptoms are a combination of depression and anxiety. In general, the earlier the symptoms appear, the longer they last. This is why it is important not to dismiss depression symptoms as temporary or unimportant, thinking that they are normal for pregnancy and will go away on their own. That old (and bad) information is based on a myth. If you experience any symptoms on the list, I recommend that you complete a depression screening tool. Each tool provides you with clear next steps depending on your score.

Depression that continues beyond pregnancy can take a few different forms. For example, after an initial bout of depression in pregnancy, about 40 percent of women experience cycles of relapse of depression. Their pattern is that they feel well for a time, and then they experience another period of depression that may last for weeks or months and range from mild to severe.

Another 40 percent of women experience persistent depression, a longer-term, low-level depression that lasts for two years or longer. Although most can continue with their daily activities, women find that the quality of their lives is affected by feeling sad and un-energized, and they often don't remember what it's like *not* to have this overriding sadness. And although the symptoms of low-level depression seem milder, the long-term effect on the baby's development is worse because it impacts the way the mother interacts with her baby for an extended period.

Self-Assessments for Depression

Like Jill, you may have had moments when you wondered whether the emotional changes you were going through were normal—or not—and if what you were experiencing was more than a mood swing. If so, you are not alone. In our work, 3 out of 4 pregnant women expressed confusion about the warning signs of depression. What I find most troubling is that their uncertainty about whether their symptoms were pregnancy related or something more prevented them from talking to their nurse or doctor about their concerns. For instance, in our work, we found that 24.5 percent of pregnant women had received a formal diagnosis of depression while *an equal number* (27.4 percent) had experienced depression symptoms but had not been diagnosed.[9] The research-based self-assessments that follow here are a first step at helping you discern what you may be struggling with so that you can move forward in the direction that serves you best.

There are a few things that you should know about self-assessment tools in general. First, like blood tests and X-rays, no assessment for depression or anxiety is 100 percent perfect. In fact, most mental health tools are about 70 percent to 85 percent accurate, which means that the results are inaccurate for 15 percent to 30 percent of women. In these cases, the most common problem is that the tool indicates that a woman *does not have* symptoms high enough to be classified as depression when in fact she *does*. (It's far less likely that the tool will identify the woman as having depression when she does not.) It's the same with a home-based pregnancy test. The tests are 98 percent to 99 percent accurate. If you test positive, you can be quite sure that you are pregnant. If you test negative, the test might be in error, and you might actually be pregnant.

If you think that you have depression, but the tool—for example, the Edinburgh Postnatal Depression Scale—indicates you don't, complete a second depression tool, such as the Patient Health Questionnaire. If you still feel convinced that the tests aren't accurate, retake them a day or two later. Don't overthink your responses—put the first answer that comes to mind. It tends to be the most unfiltered, accurate response.

Second, one assessment tool doesn't give the whole picture. For instance, you may have some mild symptoms of depression, but you have a strong support network and good coping mechanisms that are likely to help you manage your depression symptoms and prevent them from worsening. Your friend, on the other hand, may also have mild symptoms of depression but also be experiencing difficulties in her marriage, have family who live far away, and have depleted coping mechanisms, putting her at risk for worsening depression. Throughout the book, there are a variety of self-assessments to help you understand not only your symptoms (whether you have any and how high they are), but also how you cope, your risk factors, and what supports you have around you.

The Edinburgh Postnatal Depression Scale[10]

Even though the name says *postnatal*, this tool has been tested in pregnant women and found to effectively assess depression in the prenatal and postnatal periods. You can use it at any point during pregnancy and up to one year after delivery. For peace of mind, you can use it any time you want to do a self-check-in or regularly as part of your self-care, for instance, each trimester of your pregnancy, and 1 month, 3 months, 6 months, and 12 months after you have your baby.

Answer each of the ten questions, then add up the score for your total. For example, in the first question, if you answered "as much as I always could" you would give yourself a score of 0 for that question. If you answered "not quite so much now" you would give yourself a score of 1.

IN THE PAST 7 DAYS . . .	ANSWER
I have been able to laugh and see the funny side of things. As much as I always could (0) Not quite so much now (1) Definitely not so much now (2) Not at all (3)	
I have looked forward with enjoyment to things. As much as I ever did (0) Rather less than I used to (1) Definitely less than I used to (2) Hardly at all (3)	
I have blamed myself unnecessarily when things went wrong. Yes, most of the time (3) Yes, some of the time (2) Not very often (1) No, never (0)	
I have been anxious or worried for no good reason. No, not at all (0) Hardly ever (1) Yes, sometimes (2) Yes, very often (3)	

I have felt scared or panicky for no very good reason.
 	
    Yes, quite a lot (3)
    Yes, sometimes (2)
    No, not much (1)
    No, not at all (0)	

Things have been getting on top of me.
 	
    Yes, most of the time I haven't been able to cope (3)
    Yes, sometimes I haven't been coping as well as usual (2)
    No, most of the time I have coped quite well (1)
    No, I have been coping as well as ever (0)	

I have been so unhappy that I have had difficulty sleeping.
 	
    Yes, most of the time (3)
    Yes, sometimes (2)
    Not very often (1)
    No, not at all (0)	

I have felt sad or miserable.
 	
    Yes, most of the time (3)
    Yes, quite often (2)
    Not very often (1)
    No, not at all (0)	

I have been so unhappy that I have been crying.
 	
    Yes, most of the time (3)
    Yes, quite often (2)
    Only occasionally (1)
    No, never (0)	

The thought of harming myself has occurred to me.
 	
    Yes, quite often (3)
    Sometimes (2)
    Hardly ever (1)
    Never (0)	

Total Score:	

Your Results

YOUR SCORE	The Meaning of Your Score	Your Next Steps
0–8	It is unlikely that you are experiencing depression symptoms.	Continue practicing healthy lifestyle habits to support and protect your emotional health.
9–11	It is possible that you are experiencing depression symptoms.	Recheck your score in two weeks. If your score is still 9–11, begin with regular practice of the Safe and Sound Protocol (Chapter 7) and consider sharing your results with your doctor or midwife.
12–13	It is likely that you are experiencing depression symptoms in the mild to moderate range.	Implement regular practice of the Safe and Sound Protocol. In addition, make an appointment with your doctor or midwife and share your results.
14 and higher	It is likely that you are experiencing depression symptoms in the moderate to severe range.	Implement regular practice of the Safe and Sound Protocol. In addition, make an appointment with your doctor and share your results. Your doctor will likely refer you to a counsellor or psychiatrist, depending on how high your score is.

Patient Health Questionnaire[11]

This questionnaire measures depression in adults. You can use it during pregnancy, the first year after your baby is born, and beyond. Like with the Edinburgh Postnatal Depression Scale, you can use it at intervals—every trimester and after you have your baby—to get a picture of how you're doing.

Answer each of the nine questions with one of the four responses, then add up your total.

OVER THE LAST 2 WEEKS, HOW OFTEN HAVE YOU BEEN BOTHERED BY ANY OF THE FOLLOWING PROBLEMS?	Not at all	Several days	More than half the days	Nearly every day
1. Little interest or pleasure in doing things	0	1	2	3
2. Feeling down, depressed, or hopeless	0	1	2	3
3. Trouble falling or staying asleep, or sleeping too much	0	1	2	3
4. Feeling tired or having little energy	0	1	2	3
5. Poor appetite or overeating	0	1	2	3
6. Feeling bad about yourself or that you are a failure or have let yourself or your family down	0	1	2	3

7. Trouble concentrating on things, such as reading the newspaper or watching television	0	1	2	3
8. Moving or speaking so slowly that other people could have noticed. Or the opposite— being so fidgety or restless that you have been moving around a lot more than usual	0	1	2	3
9. Thoughts that you would be better off dead or hurting yourself in some way	0	1	2	3
Total Columns				
PHQ-9 Total score				

Your Results

YOUR SCORE	The Meaning of Your Score	Your Next Steps
0–4	You have minimal/no depression symptoms.	Continue practicing healthy lifestyle habits to support your emotional health.
5–9	You have mild depression symptoms.	Recheck your score in two weeks. If your score is still 5–14, share your results with your doctor or midwife. If your score is 10–14, they may refer you to a psychologist or counsellor for support. Practice the Safe and Sound Protocol regularly (Chapter 7).
10–14	You have moderate depression symptoms.	

| 15–19 | You have moderately severe depression symptoms. | Make an appointment with your doctor and share your results. Your doctor will likely refer you to a counsellor or psychiatrist. Depending on how you are managing day to day, you may also find support from taking antidepressants. Practice the Safe and Sound Protocol regularly (Chapter 7). |
| 20–27 | You have severe depression symptoms. | Make an appointment with your doctor and share your results. Your doctor will likely refer you to a counsellor or psychiatrist, depending on how high your score is. You may find support in using a combination of counselling and antidepressants. Practice the Safe and Sound Protocol regularly (Chapter 7). |

Jill's Story

At the next prenatal visit, our doctor asked me a series of questions about mood using the Edinburgh Postnatal Depression Scale. He told Josiah and me that I scored in the range of having moderate depression. We were taken aback by the diagnosis of depression, and I have to say we just weren't prepared for it. I felt guilty for not talking to the doctor earlier, thinking that I had harmed our baby. But my doctor reassured us that it was untreated depression that went on for a long time that carried risk for the baby.

I've started counselling with a great therapist, and I am working through some things that I've been hanging on to for a long time. I love that my counsellor is using neurofeedback, a brain-based approach that is helping my brain to heal from some of the things in my life that I didn't even know were impacting me. I relax in a reclining chair, she puts the cap with sensors over my hair, and I watch a movie for thirty minutes while my brain rewires itself.

I wish I had done this sooner! With every session I feel lighter, less emotionally drained, and more hopeful. I feel less anxious about labour and better prepared for our parenting journey ahead.

When you experience depression symptoms, it's easy to slide into believing that depression is part of who you are. But depression isn't a character flaw or a feature of your personality. It's a set of symptoms that you experience that is, like a fever, an indicator of something going on inside. With the decades of neurobiological research filling in the gaps, we now understand depression as a complex constellation of causes that at its heart reflects dysregulation of our brain and nervous system by difficult life circumstances.

Think about depression in the same way that you think about physical health conditions, such as diabetes. If you have diabetes, you experience high blood sugar and you need to change your diet and exercise habits to lower your blood sugar and make sure that it stays within a healthy range. If you have depression, you may experience symptoms of sadness, low self-esteem, and low energy, and you need to implement strategies to lower these symptoms and to make sure that your mental health stays within a healthy range. That simple change in the way you look at depression—as *having symptoms of depression* instead of *being depressed*—will help you to step back from your experience and see it as a challenge to be managed—not a personal flaw that you can't change.

As ever, I want to end on a hopeful note, rooted in the new paradigm of neuroscience and mental health. We don't view depression like we used to. We view it as sign of a disrupted nervous system that is protecting us, trying to help us survive life circumstances that would otherwise have overwhelmed us—and it can be healed.

CHAPTER 4

The Truth About Anxiety

Most pregnant women feel worried at some point in their journey. Pregnancy is a time of huge change, and it naturally comes with its share of concerns. When I was pregnant with my first child, I worried about whether I'd be a nurturing mother. I worried about the low-lying placenta that had been diagnosed on ultrasound. I worried about our finances and how we would manage on a reduced income during the year-long maternity leave. And when I was pregnant with our second child, I worried about how I would manage with two children under two years. Having been an only child, the deep-seated concern I didn't share with others was whether I would be able to love a second child as much as the first. Gratefully, my wise husband said that the second baby would have the love of not only his parents but of his sibling as well.

Our brains naturally interpret the ambiguity that surrounds change and transition, such as pregnancy, as a potential threat. After all, our brain's main job description is to keep us safe. When we face new experiences, a healthy brain scans our environment for signs of danger that could harm us. Although the situation may be brand new, it subconsciously looks for anything that is similar to past experiences when it perceived we were in danger. Our sense of being heightened is a sign of a well-functioning nervous system when it is proportional to the threat (a little threat, a little activation) and when it calms down after the sense of threat passes. Physically, we feel the tension pass and calm ensue. This might be described as normal worry; anxiety, on the other hand, is a persistent, non-specific sense of dread and angst that can interfere with life.[1]

In this chapter, I'll distinguish between normal worry and anxiety, and outline what the common triggers and causes of anxiety are as well as easy-to-implement strategies to reduce the risk and symptoms of anxiety. In short, anxiety is common but treatable.

What Is Anxiety and What Does It Look Like in Pregnancy?

Fatima's Story

I woke up with my teeth clenched and stomach in knots. My husband, James, was up already, and I could hear him in the kitchen making coffee. I thought about the times when I used to love the peace and calm of the mornings. But I haven't felt peace and calm for months. I let the hot tears run down my face as I thought, *What's become of me? I thought this pregnancy would be so different.*

I swung my feet over the side of the bed and walked into the shower. I stepped in, letting the warm water cascade over my already tense neck and shoulders, but I couldn't escape the dread that I felt. I replayed yesterday's day at work and evening at home. I envisioned my schedule for the day. Nothing seemed out of place, and yet the knot in my stomach tightened to a point of nausea and my fear and dread that something terrible would happen grew.

I joined James for coffee outside on our upper balcony. As I sipped my coffee in silence, he verbalized what we were both thinking: "It's getting worse, isn't it?"

I nodded, knowing that I couldn't hide it any longer. I wished I could just cry, but I only felt shame and guilt. My mother had suffered with mental health problems, and I knew what it was like to grow up in a household like that. We lived on pins and needles, never knowing when it would be a good day or a bad day.

"James, we never should have gotten pregnant. Everything is going wrong. And I know I've harmed the baby."

He reached across the table and took my hand in his. "Let's make an appointment with your midwife. I'll go with you. We'll see what can be done."

In that moment, I felt the first glimmer of promise that I'd felt in months.

—Fatima, 26 weeks

It's normal to worry. But what Fatima suffers from is a diffuse, vague sense of dread that something terrible is going to happen. It's not based on any specific event or experience, but it consumes her thoughts and emotions, causes physical symptoms (muscle tension, jaw clenching), and interferes with her life and relationships. She's suffering from anxiety.

Anxiety isn't normal. It magnifies and distorts the issue until it feels constant, insurmountable, vague, and global, washing over all areas of our lives. It's not a healthy, helpful response because, as I say to my clients, it turns the issue into a ball of yarn so entangled that you don't know where to start to solve it. When we are anxious, it is much harder to find the end of the yarn that we need to pull on to help our situation.

Previously, I shared the risk factors that are common across depression, anxiety, and stress: history of a mental health problem, stressful life events in the year before pregnancy, having a lot of conflict in your partner relationship, and not having adequate support. There are some risk factors that are also specific to anxiety, including: interpersonal violence, having a previous negative birth experience, experiencing a previous loss (e.g., miscarriage, stillbirth, abortion), and having an unplanned or unwanted pregnancy. It's not that these can't also contribute to depression, but they are more apt to relate to anxiety.

Our research and others' have also shown that as many as 60 percent of women (and men!) undergoing infertility treatment experience high degrees of anxiety. However, most research shows that this anxiety decreases significantly once women stop treatment, either voluntarily or because they become pregnant. In other words, having a hard time getting pregnant and having anxiety related to that doesn't mean that you'll continue to struggle with anxiety through your pregnancy.

The Autonomic Ladder

Like depression, anxiety is a sign of neural dysregulation, which we discussed in Chapter 1. To better understand what neural dysregulation means, let's use Dr. Deb Dana's marvelous tool: the Autonomic Ladder, which depicts our autonomic nervous system, that part of our nervous system that controls our automatic body functions such as breathing, heart rate, and responding to danger in our environment.[2, 3, 4]

Picture a ladder. At the top rung, your nervous system is in its safest state, where your ventral vagal nerve is in control. Here, you feel well. The world feels welcoming and trusting. You feel curious, engaged, open-hearted, hopeful, resourceful, and at ease. As Deb Dana says, "This is not a place where everything is wonderful or a place without problems. But it is a place where we have the ability to acknowledge distress and explore options, to reach out for support and develop organized responses."[5]

As you go down the ladder, your nervous system becomes dysregulated, perhaps by an argument with your partner or an unexpected bill in the mail. In the middle of the ladder, the first phase of dysregulation, your sympathetic nervous system becomes engaged, and you enter fight-or-flight mode because something feels dangerous and threatening. Here, the world feels unfriendly and chaotic. You feel confused, out of control, stressed, overwhelmed, and perhaps angry—and you just want to run and escape.[6] If your situation worsens—for instance, your partner refuses to speak to you for days after your conflict—you may progress even further down the ladder to the second phase of dysregulation where your dorsal vagal system is activated and you are in freeze, a place where you feel immobilized. Here, the world feels cold and empty. You feel foggy, numb, helpless, hopeless, exhausted, disconnected from others, and shut down.[7] As you and your partner remain in conflict, you may feel like you don't care, and you don't feel like ever making amends. You've given up. And so, whereas normally you might feel that you and your partner have a close and trusting relationship, in a state of dysregulation your thoughts, feelings, and behaviours can be quite different.

Our nervous system works together—the ventral vagal, sympathetic, and dorsal vagal—and we travel up and down the ladder many times in a single day. We can travel down the ladder with any encounter or situation in our lives that feels threatening to us, such as a conversation with a difficult co-worker, a car accident, a life setback, a testy comment from a neighbour, an encounter with a rude person at a store, having too much to do, and a social media post that tosses you into the comparison trap.[8] We can reach the bottom ladder (our dorsal vagal state) when we feel immobilized by workload, experience inescapable chronic pain, experience grief and loss, or are abandoned or ignored.

Our goal is to keep our nervous system regulated and at the top of the ladder in the ventral vagal state as much as possible, but persistent anxiety is a reflection of a nervous system that is dysregulated, stuck in the sympathetic activation mode and unable to be reset to perform the normal activate-rest cycle. It is a signal that your brain and nervous system have been rewired by a significant event in your life—in childhood or adulthood—that your brain interpreted as inescapable, overwhelming, uncontrollable, and threatening.[9] That dysregulation isn't limited to the brain and nervous system. As Dr. Bruce McEwen noted two decades ago, anxiety affects the function of the whole body, "including the cardiovascular, metabolic, and immune system, as well as the structure and function of the brain itself."[10]

Women are twice as likely to experience anxiety as men are, and anxiety is especially common in women aged 15 to 34—right when most women are having children.[11] So, it comes as no surprise that the latest studies indicate that more pregnant women have anxiety than we first realized.[12] As many as 20 percent to 35 percent of pregnant women experience anxiety symptoms, making it one of the leading problems that women face during the prenatal period.[13, 14]

In fact, anxiety affects roughly twice as many women as does depression during pregnancy.[15] And anxiety in pregnancy is like a double-edged sword. It increases a woman's risk of experiencing depression in pregnancy and in the postpartum period three-fold, increases her severity of mental health problems overall, and elevates her risk of postpartum anxiety. With all of this, anxiety is immensely treatable. As one of the pregnant women who joined our studies to receive help with anxiety, said, "Life can be really good!"

Symptoms of Anxiety

There are more than ten different kinds of anxiety, but all share the following signs:

- excessive and intrusive worrying, difficulty controlling the worry
- feeling overwhelmed
- irritability, anger
- fatigue, difficulty concentrating and sleeping
- a sense of fear, dread, and threat
- a tendency to see situations, people, and life negatively
- restlessness, feeling keyed up or on edge
- muscle tension
- significant distress or impairment in social, occupational, or other important areas of life as a result of the anxiety, worry, or physical symptoms

In general, your doctor would diagnose anxiety if you experienced some of these symptoms for most days over a six-month period. So, while you may be worried about your upcoming ultrasound, if your worry is short-lived and temporary (e.g., the two-week period before the ultrasound scan), then it is situational. But if you've worried about your baby's development every day for seven months, even after a positive ultrasound and regular prenatal check-ups, you may be experiencing anxiety.

It can be hard to distinguish normal worry from anxiety. In general, worry is linked to a specific situation or relationship. Your level of worry is in proportion to how challenging the situation is. It is time limited, focused on a present situation, and temporary, and it's contained to your thoughts. You are effective in creating solutions, and you don't fixate on negative outcomes.

On the other hand, anxiety is vague and diffuse. If someone were to ask you what was bothering you, it would feel like "everything." It tends to be focused on the future, anticipating the worst possible outcome. You are more bothered about the situation than is warranted. Your upset spills over across areas of your life, so that what might have begun as concern over a work situation mushrooms into fear about your upcoming ultrasound. You worry constantly—going to bed and waking in the morning with the same sense of fear and dread. You replay situations over and over in your mind and feel its physical effects (e.g., tension, stomach knots). It's hard to make decisions and think clearly, in part because the issue is so vague it is hard to find a solution.

Many women experience more than one kind of anxiety, but the three most common in pregnancy are generalized anxiety, social anxiety, and panic disorder.

Generalized anxiety looks a lot like what Fatima was experiencing. She had excessive, uncontrollable dread and foreboding, and it had lasted for months. There wasn't a specific situation she was concerned about—the global dread that she felt day after day wore her down and the anxiety-related physical symptoms added to the burden she carried.

Someone with *social anxiety* experiences the same symptoms, but they are tied to social situations. Social anxiety makes being with others painful (and exhausting) because of the relentless self-consciousness, the constant comparison, and the fear of judgment by others for what you say and do. Those with social anxiety replay conversations and behaviours, focusing on others' negative responses and scanning for their own mistakes or embarrassments. Ultimately, social anxiety holds people back from doing and saying what they really want to do because of the fear of being judged.

Panic attacks are extremely distressing experiences. They're a sign that our nervous system is in extreme dysregulation; they're sudden, heightened episodes where our brain unconsciously senses immediate danger. One pregnant woman that I counselled had nightly panic attacks where she feared that harm would come to her baby. She would wake up in terror, heart racing, breathing fast, shaking, and sweating. She literally felt like she was dying. Between attacks, she would worry about having another. And they continued for months until we started implementing parts of the Safe and Sound Protocol (Chapter 7). After a few weeks of re-regulating her nervous system with these techniques, the panic attacks simply stopped. Yes, they sometimes recur under times of extreme stress in her life, but she practices her strategies regularly again and they settle down. She is learning to keep her nervous system tuned up and regulated.

Like depression, anxiety can also be chronic. Studies from Canada, France, and Australia show that roughly 40 percent of women who develop anxiety in pregnancy and go untreated will still experience symptoms when their child is 5 years old. Decades of research illustrate that anxiety tends to have a stable trajectory—that is, if you struggle with anxiety before pregnancy, without intervention, you're likely to still struggle with it during the postpartum period and beyond—and that the combination of prenatal anxiety and depression is longer and harder to treat.

Anxiety also ranges in severity along a continuum from mild to severe. Some days, you might have quite a few symptoms and feel them strongly. Other days, you might have fewer, less intense symptoms. However, anxiety has a different pattern than depression. Depression often shows up as a one-time bout or in cycles, and even those who suffer from persistent depression experience some relief from depressive symptoms for a time.[16, 17] The natural pattern of anxiety tends to be more constant (when not treated or not treated efficaciously), and women who are first diagnosed with anxiety in pregnancy often recognize its symptoms across their lives in hindsight.

SELF-ASSESSMENT

Generalized Anxiety Disorder (GAD-7)[18] Questionnaire

The Generalized Anxiety Disorder (GAD-7) questionnaire is a brief, widely used screening tool that can help you to get a sense of whether you are struggling with anxiety. It measures your level of anxiety over the past two weeks by asking questions about the most common symptoms. You can use it any time, but I recommend completing it each trimester of your pregnancy, and after you have your baby at the 1 month, 3 months, 6 months, and 12 months milestones.

Answer each of the seven questions by selecting one of the four responses: Not at all, Several days, More than half the days, or Nearly every day. Then add up your answers for your total score.

OVER THE LAST 2 WEEKS, HOW OFTEN HAVE YOU BEEN BOTHERED BY THE FOLLOWING PROBLEMS?	Not at all	Several days	More than half the days	Nearly every day
1. Feeling nervous, anxious, or on edge	0	1	2	3
2. Not being able to stop or control worrying	0	1	2	3
3. Worrying too much about different things	0	1	2	3
4. Trouble relaxing	0	1	2	3
5. Being so restless that it is hard to sit still	0	1	2	3
6. Becoming easily annoyed or irritable	0	1	2	3
7. Feeling afraid as if something awful might happen	0	1	2	3

Your Results

YOUR SCORE	THE MEANING OF YOUR SCORE	YOUR NEXT STEPS
0–4	You have no anxiety/minimal anxiety symptoms.	Continue practicing healthy lifestyle habits to support your emotional health. Practice strategies of the Safe and Sound Protocol in Chapter 7 to keep your nervous system tuned and regulated.

5–9	You have symptoms of mild anxiety.	Recheck your score in two weeks. If your score is still 5–14, share your results with your doctor or midwife. If your score is 10–14, your doctor or midwife may refer you to a psychologist or counsellor for support. Begin to practice the Safe and Sound Protocol regularly.
10–14	You have symptoms of moderate anxiety.	
15–21	You have symptoms of severe anxiety.	Make an appointment with your doctor and share your results. Your doctor will likely refer you to a counsellor or psychiatrist. Depending on how you are managing, you may also find support from taking antidepressants. Practice the Safe and Sound Protocol regularly.

Fatima's Story

Two days later, James and I had our appointment with our midwife, Lucie. She completely understood what I was going through and asked permission to give me a series of screening questions for anxiety. After I had answered them, Lucie added my scores and explained that it showed I had anxiety symptoms.

"Fatima," she said quietly, "does this come as a surprise to you?"

"No," I replied without hesitation. "Honestly, I just feel pure relief." I had thought I'd feel more dread and fear in this appointment, but it was just the opposite.

"Many women feel the same way, Fatima," she replied. "Somehow, putting a name to a struggle helps us to define what it is and what we need to do next. It takes the fear and uncertainty out of it."

She was right. Then, Lucie looked me in the eye, and she said, "Fatima—you did nothing wrong."

The tears welled up. She had really hit a vulnerable spot.

She carried on, "Anxiety is just a sign that your nervous system is out of sync. And that can happen for lots of reasons, but they all have one thing in common—at some point you were in a situation where you felt unsafe."

Then I really started to cry. I thought of all those years growing up when I never knew whether it was a good day or a bad day. When I had to watch everything I did and said because one small wrong move would set the house into a fury of chaos and screaming.

Lucie could see that this was hard for me, and she carefully floated the idea, "What if I arrange for you to see a colleague who uses some very cutting-edge techniques to help pregnant women with anxiety? She's getting very good results."

James and I looked at each other and turned to her and nodded. Somehow, I knew in that moment it was all going to be okay.

My whole life I'd been waiting for "the pin to drop"—the moment when someone would see through me and tell me I was mentally ill. I'd seen my mother go through it. I'd seen what it did to our family. But after Lucie explained to me that I could stop this cycle from continuing, I felt hopeful. For the first time, I knew what hope felt like.

The fact is that sometimes when we're overloaded or going through a particularly tough time, anxiety is the first indication that our mental health is suffering. That warning sign is actually a good thing because it cues us to the effect of our life circumstances on our brain and nervous system. When we know what to look for, we can take steps to manage our anxiety so that it doesn't impact our daily life.

Here are some top-down pushback factors for tempering overwhelming negative thoughts and feelings:

- Be mindful. Research shows that recognizing and accepting your thoughts and feelings can help build awareness and control over your emotions, which will reduce your stress. Try sitting quietly and deep breathing to block out the noise around you and tune in to your own thoughts and feelings.
- Understand that emotions are useful. If you tend toward neuroticism, you may try to avoid experiencing negative emotions for fear that they would just make you feel worse. Understand that emotions are your body's signals and learning to listen to them is far healthier than ignoring them.
- Don't avoid difficult situations. While you might feel better in the short-term, it's more damaging long-term because you need to expose yourself to difficult circumstances to learn from them and experiment with them.

These strategies can provide temporary relief, but we'll see a decrease in rates of prenatal anxiety only when we fully embrace the neuroscientific understanding of the causes and treatment of anxiety. Rather than anxiety being viewed as an illness hinging on unhelpful thoughts, beliefs, and feelings, neuroscience research encourages us to understand it as a dysregulation of the brain and nervous system.

Rather than medication and talk therapy being the first-line choices of treatment for the symptoms of anxiety, we should be designing treatments that target the anxiety itself, i.e., the dysregulation. As we adopt new approaches for re-regulating the nervous system, I believe we will see decreasing rates of anxiety in pregnant women, and fewer infants and children plagued with the legacy of intergenerational distress.

CHAPTER 5

The Truth About Stress

Everybody has stress. Stress is normal. Stress is good for you. Stress helps you perform at your best.

We hear these statements all the time, and each is true. But they tell only one side of the story—that of *eustress*, or beneficial stress. Many of us have normalized our experience of stress and thus minimized the physical and emotional consequences of *dis*tress, or what scientists call *toxic stress*.

Our research shows that roughly 13 percent of pregnant women have a high level of stress that affects their health and well-being; another 50 percent have moderate levels of stress that make daily living hard and reduce their ability to experience their pregnancy in the way they had hoped.[1] Together, these statistics tell us that 2 out of every 3 pregnant women struggle with stress that significantly affects their daily lives.

Of the three most common emotional health challenges in pregnancy—depression, anxiety, and stress—stress has been most extensively researched, primarily because it's easier to study stress in animals than anxiety and depression and much of the early work was animal based. We know more about how stress affects us physically and emotionally—and how it affects the baby—than any other form of emotional distress. For more than fifty years, researchers have published data on the consequences of high stress in pregnancy, from studying rats and zebrafish in laboratories to baboons in the African wild, and finally human pregnancy. But this information has been unacceptably slow to trickle down into applicable, clinical care. For example, rarely do our practitioners ask pregnant women about their levels of stress.

This chapter will describe the neurobiology of stress as the dysregulation of the nervous system and provide tools that you can use to assess your degree of stress so that you can manage it and stay at a level of healthy, beneficial eustress.

What Is Stress and What Does It Look Like in Pregnancy?

Margaret's Story

"And so, unfortunately, we can't approve your promotion. Just get a little more experience under your belt and we'll re-evaluate where you're at in six months."

I heard the words my supervisor spoke, but I was stunned. My mouth went dry, and I could barely speak. I just nodded my head and tried to walk at a measured pace out of my supervisor's office, even though every fibre of my being wanted to run.

Six months! He didn't know I was pregnant and that I didn't have six months to get more experience—or to prove myself *again*. It was so unfair. I deserved a promotion. I thought of all the times I'd been passed over, always with the same advice— "Get more experience. Another six months."

Instead of going back to my office, I went into the bathroom. I didn't want others to see me. I splashed my face with cold water and then started to cry. I didn't know what more I could do to get this promotion—I'd exhausted all my possibilities. My mind raced, I was going to be stuck here forever, in this dead-end job. I needed this to happen before my maternity leave, but now it will be at least two years down the road. Did I really need this job? But if I left before my maternity leave, I wouldn't get my top-up, and we'd be financially strapped. There was no way out!

That night, as I told my husband, Peter, about my meeting with my supervisor and how I'd been passed over for a promotion again, the knots grew in my stomach. I felt like it was all going downhill, and there was nothing I could do to stop it. I felt powerless to make any impact on this terrible situation.

"It's okay," he replied matter-of-factly. "It will happen when you get back. The timing will be better."

I raised my voice. "No! It won't be! If it doesn't happen now, it never will!" I was irritated at him that he didn't get it.

"Mags, we need to take a step back here and look at this realistically. If you got the promotion now, you'd be working day and night until the baby is born. You'd be under intense pressure. You wouldn't have time to do all the things you want to get ready for the baby."

I knew he was making sense. But the sense of threat that I carried wasn't going away.

I slept poorly, waking every few hours. In the morning, I reached out to my friend, Anne, knowing that I needed her professional counselling wisdom.

—Margaret, 24 weeks

Margaret was experiencing a significant stressor in her life, and it catapulted her brain, nervous system, and body into a full-blown stress response. In short, stressors are *things that we find stressful because we see them as inherently dangerous or threatening*.

Every stressor is different in terms of the mental, emotional, and physical demands it places on us. Ultimately, the specific type of stressor is unimportant. The key piece is that it has an activating influence on us *because our brain interprets it as dangerous*. Our brains are constantly scanning our environment for signs of potential danger—a process called *neuroception*—whether we are resting, making supper, working at the office, having a conversation with a friend, or driving around our neighbourhood.[2] Our reactions to stressors happen on many levels, but the main impact is on our brain and nervous system, and once these systems are triggered, they activate a flood of biochemical and physiological changes that ultimately filter down to our thoughts and actions.

According to Dr. Bruce McEwen, the brain is the key organ affected by stress.[3] That's because stress is first detected in deeply buried parts of our brain, including a small, almond-shaped structure called the amygdala, which acts as our body's main threat and danger detector. The amygdala is like command central that interprets all these things as either safe or threatening and dangerous. If it judges something we see or experience as threatening, it becomes activated and, like a good commander, launches a threat response. It sends signals to our other organs to prepare our body to (1) stay and fight the danger, (2) run away from it, or (3) play dead until the threat passes us by—three actions that are intended to keep us safe.

Our stress system is called the *hypothalamic-pituitary-adrenal (HPA) axis* and is a highly organized system that fans out across our body to quicken our thinking so that we can make rapid decisions; ramp up our heartbeat, breathing, and blood pressure so that we can act quickly; enhance our immune response so that we are better protected if injured; and decrease all the body functions that we don't need in an emergency—like emptying our bladder. If these strategies don't remove us from the danger, then our systems shut down and we literally become immobilized ("play dead").

Thanks to the work of Dr. McEwen, we now understand that there are three different kinds of stress: good or normal stress (eustress), tolerable stress, and toxic stress.[4]

Good stress is what you experience when you face a challenge in your daily life and manage it with success. It is mild or moderate in intensity and short-lived so that physiological responses (such as increased heart rate or breathing, a sense of agitation) are brief. For instance, you might be a bit worried about your upcoming fetal ultrasound, but you take steps to talk to a friend and are reassured that it will be fine. You had resources, used them, and they were sufficient to help you reduce your stress. This is the kind of stress that produces resilience because it gives our nervous system the opportunity to practice the normal pattern of brief activation of the nervous system followed by deactivation and calm. As children, our brain and nervous system learn resilience when we have a responsive adult help us manage day-to-day stressors, such as going to a new place, so that our nervous system learns to re-regulate and move back into a calm state.[5]

Tolerable stress is when you experience a challenging life situation, your brain and nervous system are activated, and you experience the mobilization of all the other components of the stress response (your immune, inflammatory, and metabolic systems). However, you are still able to manage the stressor well because you have good coping skills and internal resources, such as reaching out to your support network and neurobiologically regulating practices.

Tolerable stress is limited in time and intensity because the stressor is itself time limited or because we have sufficient resiliency to keep its effects contained within a manageable window. For example, after having your ultrasound, your doctor says that there are some views that are not clear or she thinks she sees something a bit off, and she wants you to have a second ultrasound. Although you feel significant stress, you manage it by talking to your partner, asking your doctor questions so that you have all the information, and taking time to walk outside and talk with a trusted friend. You practice deep breathing regularly throughout the day and listen to calming harp music. As a result, your stress level stays within a reasonable, manageable level.

Toxic stress arises when you experience a challenging life circumstance, and your brain and nervous system experience significant dysregulation that is frequent or prolonged, but you can't manage it well because the situation is so overwhelming that it is beyond your capacity to manage. For instance, you unexpectedly get laid off from your job only two months before your due date. Rather than working through this difficult situation and creating a plan for managing it, you just can't draw upon your internal and external resources effectively. You imagine the worst possible outcomes, such as you will not be able to get another job, you and your partner will not be able to pay your bills, and you will be financially destitute during your maternity leave. You struggle to adjust to your new situation and continue to feel high stress. Toxic stress can be reduced to tolerable stress (and good stress) with the presence and support of a safe, trusted relationship and regular implementation of key strategies for re-regulating the nervous system.

Toxic stress is the most damaging, physically and emotionally. Sometimes it happens because the things we face are overwhelming. Sometimes it happens because we've been facing a difficult situation for a prolonged time, and our internal bodily checks and balances are getting worn down. When our bodies and minds become depleted by the stress load, our ability to implement healthy brain practices suffers. We may have disrupted sleep, eat poorly, cut back on exercise, and self-isolate from trusted friends—all of which takes joy and energy from our lives and can put us at risk for developing depression and anxiety symptoms.

Each of us reacts to different stressors, and our responses to those stressors are unique. Dr. Jack Shonkoff, director of the Center on the Developing Child (Harvard University), says it best: "The source, type, or number of adverse experiences does not define toxic stress . . . it is the magnitude, duration, and timing of the biological and behavioural disruptions that lead to increased risk of chronic illness later in life."[6] And the magnitude of a stressful experience is personal. You may feel stressed about your upcoming ultrasound, while your friend feels fine about hers. You may react to your physician telling you that your blood pressure is slightly elevated by accepting the news and asking your doctor about next steps, while your pregnant co-worker responds with alarm and tears. Being more reactive as opposed to being intentionally responsive is tougher on us physically and emotionally, which is why managing our responses is key.[7]

How is it that two people can interpret the same situation so differently, experiencing responses at the opposite ends of the stress continuum? To answer that question, we need to dig down a little in the neurobiology of stress. Our brain and nervous system are beautifully designed to detect danger long before it ever registers in the thinking centres of our brain. They gather and interpret data from all our senses—sight, smell, touch (skin sensations), hearing, and taste. If any of these senses detects something that even remotely mimics a past threat, our brain and nervous system will interpret the current situation as danger and send chemical signals to our body to mobilize the chemical and physiological "troops" to position our body to react and get to safety.

This marvelous system, intended to protect us from danger and keep us safe, is primed by early experience. When you were a young child (especially 1 to 6 years of age), your brain and nervous system were in the midst of a sensitive period, being actively refined to "optimally fit" the environment you lived in.[8] For example, if you were raised in a home with physical abuse, your brain would be specifically primed to react to loud noises and arguments or any other sign that a beating was imminent. Any situations in adulthood that remind your nervous system of that early environment become stressors, triggering your brain and nervous system to react with the same strategies they refined when you first experienced that stressful, overwhelming situation. So, if you were hospitalized as a child and you didn't have the calming influence of a safe and supportive adult, the very thought of a prenatal amniocentesis might be triggering for you because you perceive the situation as overwhelming and threatening.

Are these conscious triggers? Often not. We may not directly connect early experiences to adult reactions. But working with a therapist can uncover them and foster healing so that they lose their triggering power.

Circumstances and events that wire our brain and nervous system to react to present-day events don't occur only in childhood; in fact, the basis of traumatic stress as we now understand it is any situation (in childhood or adulthood) that continues to affect us in our daily lives. Overall, we are more affected by situations when they tip our brain and nervous system into a state of dysregulation, generally because they:

- are severe
- feel inescapable

- are long-lasting, carrying on for weeks and months versus hours and minutes
- cluster together (e.g., several life challenges occur at the same time)
- follow one after another without a break in between
- are interpersonal or related to our significant relationships
- affect our lives significantly (e.g., your house floods versus your community has flooding)
- are unexpected, such as an unplanned job loss
- feel uncontrollable, such as the COVID-19 pandemic

On the flip side, we tend to manage better when our brain and nervous system stay regulated because the situations:

- are short-lived
- happen one at a time (or if they happen together, we feel we can manage)
- are less personally important to us and don't impact our relationships with our significant others
- provide some warning ahead of time
- feel manageable and controllable

Symptoms of Toxic Stress

In his book *Why Zebras Don't Get Ulcers*, Dr. Robert Sapolsky talks about our stress system's function to protect us and keep us safe.[9] He vividly brings it all down to a predator chasing a mammal for what he calls three minutes of screaming terror on the savannah—where he, tongue in cheek, says that one way or another, it's all over with.

The design of our stress system to be all out and then over, as in a life-or-death situation, is overkill for most of the stressful situations we face in our modern world. Today, our most impactful stressors are usually social in nature where, as Sapolsky says, our biggest problems are each other. Conflict with our partners. The one person at work who just rubs us the wrong way every time we see them. The neighbour who we just can't make sense of. The family situation that creates heartache. Stress can also be caused by comparing ourselves to others (which seems to be even more of a challenge when we're pregnant), feeling or being rejected by others, and feeling or being socially alone and unsupported.[10]

When a situation causes our stress system to kick in, but for only a brief time before it kicks out again, like a car engine revving then slowing down again, our stress is normal or tolerable. The challenge, whether personal or professional, doesn't affect our sleep, or if it does, we're able to calm our mind and fall back to sleep. We're better able to handle the situation because we have satisfying relationships; they may be imperfect, but in general, they're strong enough to work through difficulties. Life isn't always easy, but you still feel a sense of purpose and aren't overwhelmed by the situation.

When we experience toxic stress, however, our stress system kicks in and stays activated for a long period (days, weeks, or months), which depletes our energy and affects our immune response, making us more prone to illness. We may sleep poorly, either because it takes a long time to fall asleep, we wake up several times in the night, or we wake up early and cannot get back to sleep. Other symptoms of toxic stress include feeling:

- tired all the time and like you don't have energy
- nervous or anxious
- irritable

- sad or depressed
- demoralized

Under toxic stress, we also feel overwhelmed by daily life. We often find it hard to think logically about the situation because our emotions overtake us and our thoughts focus on the worst possible outcomes. We might think only in extremes; for example, if it's a work-related stressor, we might think our only choices are to quit or stay in the job.

Our perception of a situation plays a key role in our stress response, and thus our brain health.[11] Earlier, I shared my picture of our brain as a lighthouse that is constantly scanning and reading its environment for danger. At a very cellular and molecular level, our bodies are also scanning for danger with over 100,000 proteins that reside on every cell in our body. As Dr. Bruce Lipton describes, when these proteins read our environment accurately for danger, our body reacts and we survive.[12] When they misread the environment, our body reacts when it doesn't have to (e.g., a mismatch between the presence of environmental danger and our body's response), and we experience bodily damage, the effects of a stress system turned against itself.

Self-Assessments for Stress

There are two kinds of stress questionnaires to help you assess your degree of stress. The first, the Recent Life Changes Questionnaire, judges your level of stress based on the number and impact of potentially stressful life events you experienced in the past year. The second, the Perceived Stress Scale, assesses your level of stress based on how you are personally affected by significant life circumstances.

The Recent Life Changes Questionnaire[13]

Typical life events can act as risk factors for high stress and illness in our lives. The Recent Life Changes Questionnaire measures the number of stressful life events you experienced in the past year and their impact on your mental health and emotional well-being. A year with a lot of difficult life situations often can be a blur, and you may not see the level of impact that the pile of situations has on you until you take the time to reflect on your experiences.

You can complete this questionnaire any time, but I recommend at least once during your pregnancy and 6 to 12 months later. Check off each life situation that you experienced in the past year, then add up the Life Impact Rating (last column of table). If you experienced an event twice, double your score.

YOUR LIST	RECENT LIFE CHANGES	LIFE IMPACT RATING
Work		
	Change to a new type of work	51
	Change in your work hours or conditions	35
	More work responsibilities	29
	Fewer work responsibilities	21
	A promotion	31
	A demotion	42
	A transfer	32

	Trouble with your boss	29
	Trouble with your co-workers	35
	Trouble with those you supervise	35
	Other work troubles	28
	Major business readjustment	60
	Retirement	52
	Laid off	68
	Fired	79
	Took a course to help work	18
Home and Family		
	Move within same city or town	25
	Move to different town, city, or province	47
	Major change in living conditions	42
	Change in family get-togethers	25
	Major change in health or behaviour of a family member	55
	Marriage	50
	Pregnancy	67
	Miscarriage or abortion	65
	Birth of a child	66
	Adoption of a child	65

	Relative moves in with you	59
	Spouse begins or stops work	46
	Child leaves home for college or marriage	41
	Child leaves home for other reasons	45
	Change in arguments with spouse	50
	Problems with relatives/in-laws	38
	Parents divorce	59
	A parent remarries	50
	Separation from spouse due to work	53
	Separation from spouse due to marital difficulties	79
	Divorce	96
	Birth of a grandchild	43
	Death of a spouse	119
	Death of a child	123
	Death of a parent	100
	Death of a sibling	102
Health		
	An illness or injury that kept you in bed for more than a week or sent you to the hospital	74
	An illness or injury that was less serious than above	44

Major dental work	26
Major change in eating habits	27
Major change in sleeping habits	26
Major change in your usual type and/or amount of recreation	28
Personal and Social	
Change in personal habits	26
Beginning or ending school	38
Change in school or college	35
Change in political beliefs	24
Change in religious beliefs	29
Change in social activities	27
Vacation	24
New close personal relationship	37
Engagement to marry	45
Girlfriend or boyfriend problems	39
Sexual difficulties	44
An accident	48
"Falling out" of a close personal relationship	47
Minor violation of the law	20
Being held in jail	75

	Major decision about immediate future	51
	Major personal achievement	36
	Death of a close personal friend	70
Financial		
	Major loss of income	60
	Major increase in income	38
	Investment and/or credit difficulties	56
	Loss/damage to personal property	43
	Major purchase	37
	Moderate purchase	20
	Foreclosure on a mortgage or loan	58
Your total score:		

Your Results

All life challenges have the potential to be life's teaching tools and opportunities to build resilience and capacity for handling hard things. That's why even good things, such as getting engaged, have a certain number of points attached to them. But as I've shared, multiple life challenges occurring all at once can threaten our ability to cope. That is why for this tool, the higher your score, the greater your risk. If your twelve-month score is 500 or more, you may have a high risk of developing a major stress-related mental or physical illness, depending on how well you cope with these stressful situations. This is also true if you've completed the questionnaire based on the last six months and your score is 300 or more.

In the past, we would have said, "We can't always control our external circumstances, but we can change our attitude toward them." And that is half true. With the foundation of neuroscience we now have to draw upon, a more accurate statement is, "We can't always control our external circumstances, but we can change how our brain and nervous system respond to them."[14] And when our nervous system is regulated, then we have the capacity to think differently.

The Perceived Stress Scale[15, 16]

But it's more than just being in the middle of a stressful life event that matters. The more important issue is how it affects you. Think about it like an earthquake. Your partner might experience "stress tremors" when he is in a situation that measures 6 on a scale of 1 to 10, but you feel them when you face a situation that measures a 2. You feel more bothered about situations that other people might seem to handle with little effort.

The Perceived Stress Scale measures your perception of stress, or the degree to which you are affected by stressful life experiences in the last month. It's based on the idea that although people may experience the same difficult situation, each will respond uniquely. You can complete this check-in anytime, though I recommend filling it out each trimester and every 3 to 4 months after you've had your baby.

Answer each question with how often you had that particular experience in the last month, and then add up your responses to find your total score.

QUESTION	Never	Almost Never	Some-times	Fairly Often	Very Often
In the last month, how often have you been upset because of something that happened unexpectedly?	0	1	2	3	4
In the last month, how often have you felt that you were unable to control the important things in your life?	0	1	2	3	4
In the last month, how often have you felt nervous and stressed?	0	1	2	3	4
In the last month, how often have you felt confident about your ability to handle your personal problems?	4	3	2	1	0
In the last month, how often have you felt that things were going your way?	4	3	2	1	0
In the last month, how often have you found that you could not cope with all the things that you had to do?	0	1	2	3	4
In the last month, how often have you been able to control irritations in your life?	4	3	2	1	0
In the last month, how often have you felt that you were on top of things?	4	3	2	1	0

In the last month, how often have you been angered because of things that were outside of your control?	0	1	2	3	4
In the last month, how often have you felt difficulties were piling up so high that you could not overcome them?	0	1	2	3	4
Your Score:					

Your Results

YOUR SCORE	THE MEANING OF YOUR SCORE	YOUR NEXT STEPS
0–13	You have been experiencing low stress in the past month.	Continue to manage your stress through lifestyle, good coping strategies, and brain health techniques like the Safe and Sound Protocol (Chapter 7).
14–26	You have been experiencing moderate stress in the past month.	Moderate stress, if not managed well, can turn into high stress—or become chronic, ongoing stress that increases your risk of anxiety and/or depression. Now is the time to reduce your stress level so that it does not worsen. See Chapter 7 for brain health strategies.
27–40	You have been experiencing high stress in the past month.	High levels of stress place you at greater risk for anxiety and depression and are likely impacting your home and work life. Practice stress management strategies and brain health techniques, but also consider sharing your results with your partner or a trusted friend or family member. It can be helpful to work with a counsellor about how to manage your neurobiological regulation and/or control your life circumstances in a way that doesn't continue to increase your stress.

Margaret's Story

The next day, I met Anne at a local shop for coffee and told her about the meeting with my supervisor.

She looked me straight in the eye and said quietly, "You feel betrayed."

"Yes," I said quickly. "That's exactly it. I thought they valued my work. I thought I had a place in the organization." I could feel my anger growing.

Anne could tell. Right in the middle of the coffee shop, she said, "Close your eyes. Take a deep breath. Hold it for four, three, two, one. And let it out slowly. Keep going."

I'd heard Anne talk about deep breathing before and how it calms the brain. Then she took me through a few more exercises, which she recommended I do regularly. At the end, I felt some relief. I didn't feel agitated. I didn't feel trapped. I could think more clearly. Then, Anne and I were able to talk strategically about career planning. I knew I was going to be okay and there would be a solution.

Margaret was experiencing tolerable stress, and when she reached out to her husband and friend and employed deep breathing and other calming strategies, her stress level decreased, and she was able to begin to solve her work problem. As children, we build the ability to manage tolerable stress when we have at least one responsive adult who provides a sense of security and therefore helps our brain-based responses to stay within a manageable realm.[17]

Surrounding yourself with safe people is a key pushback factor that calms and grounds our nervous system. Dr. Henry Cloud says a safe person is "a person who accepts me just like I am. A person who loves me no matter how I am being or what I do. A person whose influence develops my ability to love and be responsible."

Having little social support is one of the biggest risks for prenatal depression and anxiety. Years of research affirms that getting support from trusted friends and family is one of the best things you can do to reduce your risk of depression and anxiety and to lower your stress and even prevent these mental health problems. Cultivate safe connections, the kind Dr. Cloud talks about. Go for a walk with a trusted friend. Meet a friend for coffee. Share your heart. Give and receive. Ask for what you need. It's like watering your soul.

An effective bottom-up pushback factor for stress is resilience, and one way to build it is to reframe your experience. You might not be able to change what's happened (or is happening) in your life, but you can manage your response to it. In fact, the defining feature of people who describe their lives as satisfying and rich is not the absence of difficult situations—it's that they have learned how to cope with life's challenges. They have reframed the meaning of the situation from stressful and difficult to an opportunity of growth and learning. This isn't the easy path! Reactions to major transitions often involve fear, loss, uncertainty, overwhelm, disillusionment, doubt, and confusion. Reframing all of this to something that seems good takes ongoing effort. And it won't be effective unless you've first regulated your nervous system.

Some questions that you can ask yourself to move you from stress, fear, and confusion to a place of possibility and growth are:

- What is made possible because of this situation?
- What are your best hopes in this situation?

- What is already working in the right direction? What are signs of progress?
- If you could fast forward a week or a month, what would you want to be different? What is one step that you could take to move toward that?

Chronic Stress

I've talked about stress having a good side. When we feel our body tense up or feel a knot in our stomach, it's a signal that all is not well. Our bodies are designed to detect, react, and calm down again—all within seconds or minutes. But when you experience stressors for days, weeks, or months, or stressful situations pile up, your stress system stays ramped up on high alert. Dr. Bruce McEwen calls this *allostatic load*, and it creates wear and tear on our body.[18]

Researchers now know that wear and tear comes in the form of cardiovascular, immunity, inflammation, and metabolic health problems that can result in infection, diabetes, high blood pressure, and obesity. In addition to chronic stress increasing our risk for physical symptoms, it increases our chances of depression and anxiety. Studies show that as many as 80 percent of individuals with depression and anxiety had high stress before that evolved into symptoms of depression and anxiety. In a study in the US of more than 91,000 pregnant women, those who experienced high stress in pregnancy were five times more likely to experience postpartum depression.[19, 20] Our studies also show that women's stress tends to be long-lasting, where (without intervention) women who experience high stress in pregnancy continue to have high levels of stress even three years after their child is born.

Just as prenatal depression and anxiety can affect the baby through fetal programming, so, too, can prenatal toxic stress. While we don't have the whole picture of how prenatal stress affects the baby, we do know that normally about 10 percent of the total amount of the stress hormone that mothers naturally produce and that is in her blood crosses the placenta and enters the baby's blood system. When a mother experiences stress in pregnancy, the placenta becomes less healthy, allowing the mother's stress chemicals that normally should not cross the placental barrier to flow to the baby.[21] The baby is exposed to more stress chemicals, and the baby's brain and nervous system become rewired so that it interprets even innocent situations as threat and danger. The baby's brain and nervous system become physically reprogrammed so that it is better prepared to react to danger when he/she is born because his intrauterine environment is telling him that his/her world is not a safe place.

For well over fifty years, researchers have been studying the consequences of prenatal stress on babies and they have found that high stress in pregnancy has the potential to affect the child by increasing the chances of:

- depression and anxiety
- personality disorder
- attention deficit/hyperactivity disorder (ADHD)
- autism spectrum disorder (ASD)
- developmental delays (gross and fine motor skills, cognitive skills, shorter attention span, speech and language delay)
- difficult temperament (baby is harder to soothe and more reactive)
- emotional dysregulation (child reacts easily and calms slowly)
- behavioural problems[22]

In a recent study of more than 1,500 women of various ethnicities from all over the United States, women who experienced more negative life events, a greater negative impact of life events, and a higher perceived stress birthed children who had a higher chance of developmental delay.[23] While each of these factors impacted the child, the one that had the greatest risk was *perceived* stress. Our situation matters, but how our brain and nervous system interpret and react to our situation matters more.

But as we've discussed in Chapter 1, the epigenetic tags formed through fetal programming are not permanent. These tags can be added on *and* taken off as we face adversity throughout our lives because our brains are resilient—built to overcome insults that happen inside and outside of the mother's womb. Even when babies are exposed to high prenatal stress, a safe relationship with their parents can reduce their chances of experiencing developmental and emotional problems. For instance, a study of more than 10,000 families in the United Kingdom found that when 17-month-old infants were *insecurely* attached to their mothers (who had high prenatal stress), they showed cognitive delays. But when infants were securely attached to their mothers (who also all had high prenatal stress), they showed normal cognitive development. All the infants' mothers experienced high stress during pregnancy. The difference was the safe and responsive maternal relationship *after* the baby was born.

As Dr. Jack Shonkoff notes, the best thing that you can do for your child is build a responsive relationship, which regulates their nervous system and helps them to feel safe.[24] Imagine feeling safe every day. It would be an environment you could thrive and be your best in! You can build a secure attachment with your baby by:

- looking your baby in the eyes and talking to him
- responding to her cries promptly with comfort
- speaking in a warm, soothing voice
- holding and cuddling your baby
- reading stories to your baby
- playing with your baby

All these strategies are natural impulses for a mother. I see this on our sheep farm when, after giving birth, an ewe's voice changes to a low, soothing sound that she uses to speak to her baby lambs. She nudges them while they are feeding to bring them to her side for warmth. When they are out of sight, she calls them, and they come running to her.

Similarly, women innately know how to be what their infant needs.

Toxic stress has always been recognized as dysregulation of the nervous system. And, of depression, anxiety, and stress, the linkages and pathways between prenatal stress and negative child outcomes are best understood. Yet rarely do prenatal care providers ask women about their level of stress or offer support for toxic stress. Indeed, in his recent book, *The Myth of Normal,* medical doctor Gabor Maté delineates the same lack of essential mental health care, concluding that we're asking the wrong questions when we separate out physical illness from what is going on in people's lives.[25] My hope is that bringing the pervasive consequences of stress on women, babies, and families to the forefront presses health care providers to give pre-emptive, instead of reactive, mental health care and arms women and their families with resources to interrupt the cycle of toxic stress.

CHAPTER 6

Under the Radar

Let me begin with a story. When we bought our sheep farm, we knew we wanted to lamb, which meant we needed to get our ewes pregnant. That involved a ram, a ram harness, and several YouTube videos to figure out how to tie on the ram harness with its block of coloured crayon strapped to his underside. The idea was that once the ram mounted a ewe, he would leave behind a large, coloured circle on their bottoms or mark on their backs—evidence of the romantic interlude. We had seen pictures in our Facebook sheep groups of ewes lined up at a hay feeder showing off the symmetrical, brightly coloured sheep bottoms, as shepherds rubbed their hands in glee at the number of lambs they would see just a short five months later.

But as Dodge Ram got into action, we quickly learned it wasn't that easy. Did that pale red side swipe on Gwendolyn's right hip count as being marked? What about that orange colour on the tip of Libbie Loo's tail? Did that mean she was marked and would delight us with baby lambs in the spring? Needless to say, I was frustrated. It seemed so simple. Where were all the large painted butt circles?

We think that screening for depression, anxiety, and stress is as clear and definitive as large red butt circles on pregnant sheep, when in reality, it just isn't. Two types of mental health problems—comorbidities (when two or more mental health problems co-occur) and sub-clinical symptoms (that don't show up on assessment tools)—make it difficult.

Combined depression, anxiety, and stress look and feel different, which is why there is a section in this chapter that will help you to know what to look for. You'll also find this chapter helpful in understanding that sometimes depression, anxiety, and stress carry on beyond pregnancy, and whether you might be at risk for continuing symptoms.

Comorbidities: Combinations of Depression, Anxiety, and Stress

Both prenatal care providers and pregnant women presume that depression, anxiety, and stress occur separately. But many pregnant women and new mothers experience depression, anxiety, and/or stress symptoms *at the same time.* In fact, our research and others show that 30 percent to 60 percent of women experience both depression and anxiety simultaneously.[1, 2]

Why do the majority of women experience a combination? Most research suggests that the same brain areas and underlying biological processes are involved in depression, anxiety, and stress, and that is why there is some symptom overlap. In fact, this is driving the advent of transdiagnostic approaches, treatments that target the common underlying causes of symptoms of depression, anxiety, and stress. From a neurobiological perspective, this makes sense. Dysregulation of the nervous system manifests as symptoms of depression, anxiety, and stress.

Depression, anxiety, and stress are the most common combination in pregnancy, and the most frequent symptom pattern of this triad includes nervousness, excessive and/or uncontrollable worry, being easily fatigued, and having trouble sleeping (even more than usual!). Women also describe themselves as being overwhelmed with sentiments of shame, failure, and inadequacy, feeling angry, having a racing mind, and being irritable and unable to relax. But there is a lot of individual variation, and you might have any combination of symptoms.

Combinations of depression, anxiety, and stress are frequently underdiagnosed (and undertreated). Either women are not assessed by their practitioners for mental health problems at all, or they are checked only for symptoms of depression (because the general focus is on postpartum depression). Often, it's the anxiety component that isn't detected. And this is where advocating for yourself during prenatal appointments, ensuring that your provider doesn't dismiss your symptom profile, and the self-assessments in the earlier chapters can help. This kind of early detection is important, because the longer you wait to get help, the longer it can take for your symptoms to get better.

Knowing that you are experiencing a combined depression-anxiety can also help explain why you feel the way you do. Often, people with any combination of depression, anxiety, and stress feel worse than those who have only one, and they have a harder time functioning in their daily lives. The combined symptoms seem to have a more intense effect. For instance, one study showed that pregnant women with depression alone reported having healthier social relationships, spending more time in leisure activities, and experiencing greater life satisfaction overall than women who struggle with both depression and anxiety. In short, women with combined symptoms struggle more in their daily lives.

The other important thing to know about combined symptoms is that they can last longer and be harder to treat than either depression, anxiety, or stress on their own. For instance, one study showed that 60 percent of women who engaged in treatment for depression alone experienced complete remission of their symptoms, whereas only 21 percent of those with a combination of depression, anxiety, and stress symptoms experienced the same degree of relief. In other words, depression alone is less severe and resolves faster than a depression-anxiety-stress combination. Also, the treatment approach is often different when depression, anxiety, and stress occur together compared to when any of them occur alone. While this information may be hard to hear, it can help to set your expectations for how you manage your symptoms and the course of recovery.

Stress, Anxiety, and Postpartum Depression

In many cases, the symptoms of anxiety and stress are the first to appear and last to leave, so that the first change you notice is heightened worry over things that you normally wouldn't be as concerned about. If you experience high stress or anxiety, your risk of developing depression jumps by two to six times.

This is important because our research and others' show that women who experience anxiety and stress *during* pregnancy are much more likely to experience prenatal and postpartum depression and anxiety.[3, 4] In fact, prenatal anxiety is the biggest risk factor for postpartum depression, with as many as 60 percent of women with prenatal anxiety going on to develop postpartum depression (versus 12 percent of women who develop postpartum depression but never experienced anxiety). Knowing that anxiety and stress increase your risk of depression and anxiety after delivery is good rationale for early identification and putting into place during pregnancy the timely support strategies (self-management or professional) that can help lower your risk of postpartum depression and anxiety.

Sub-clinical Symptoms: Under the Radar

Sub-clinical symptoms of depression, anxiety, and stress also make it difficult to identify—and treat—mental health problems. You'll notice in many of the assessments in this book, there is a table with ranges of scores that guide you to understand your level of distress and next steps. Sub-clinical symptoms are just below the range of concerning scores. For instance, on the Edinburgh Postnatal Depression Scale, a score of 9 or greater corresponds to depression. If you scored an 8, in the sub-clinical domain, your prenatal provider's response might be (but probably shouldn't be): You're fine!

But our team has studied sub-clinical symptoms and been alarmed by its characteristics. In many ways, I am most concerned about women with sub-clinical symptoms for the following four reasons.

First, sub-clinical symptoms of depression, anxiety, and stress that are under the radar or barely below the cut-off to be called full-blown depression or anxiety can continue for months and years. They still impact women's daily lives. In fact, women who have long-lasting, sub-clinical symptoms of depression or anxiety tend to have lives that look very much like women with moderate or severe symptoms. Almost 2 in 3 have had depression at some point in the past. Their relationships are affected. They have a tough time connecting with their partner and friends. They feel inadequate and don't feel a sense of joy in their lives. They feel physically exhausted and depleted and mentally worn down.

Second, the number of women with sub-clinical symptoms is much larger than those with severe symptoms. Our studies and others' show that 30 percent to 40 percent of pregnant women have sub-clinical anxiety or depression, or both.[5]

Third, women with severe symptoms are more likely to have their symptoms noticed and to access treatment. However, women with sub-clinical symptoms don't receive the same care and monitoring. Their symptoms can either get better (their symptoms decrease) or they get worse (their symptoms increase in number and intensity, and they cross the threshold into depression, anxiety, or a combination). Because women and their health practitioners don't generally register low-lying symptoms as a problem, women don't have the opportunity to manage these symptoms—before they worsen.

Fourth, sub-clinical symptoms of depression or anxiety that carry on for months or years have almost the same impact on children's development and mental health as severe symptoms, as noted in Chapter 1. When I realized this, it shifted the whole nature of our team's work. Now, in addition to advocating for routine prenatal mental health screening, we educate women and their families on the facts of sub-clinical symptoms.

The key takeaway here is that you don't have to have *severe* symptoms for you or your child to be significantly affected by prenatal depression, anxiety, or stress. What is more critical than how *high* your symptoms are is *how long* your symptoms go on for. The main effects of prenatal depression, anxiety, and stress on child health and development occur when symptoms have been long-lasting. How long? No one knows for certain.

There is hope that new neuroscience tools can truncate the length of time you spend with symptoms of depression, anxiety, and stress, supplanting them with healthy processes of neuroplasticity that are ultimately passed on intergenerationally to your children's children. Indeed, it is my hope that this book inspires women and health care providers to turn our focus from researching the effects of chronic depression, anxiety, and stress to adopting brain-based techniques that disrupt chronic, long-lasting symptoms and benefit mothers and babies.

CHAPTER 7

Building Brain Health

When it comes to mental health, we're guilty of applying the same medical model used with physical illness and disease: calling interventions treatments, naming sufferers patients, and treating the brain as a sick organ. With the vast foundation of neuroscience accessible to us today, we can change our thinking from *treatment of mental illness* to *building brain health*. Many of these strategies will be new to you, but I believe they will become mainstream interventions as our knowledge of how the brain heals itself increases and we find ways to actively foster its neuroplastic capabilities.

As we now know, depression, anxiety, and stress have the same causal foundation: dysregulation of the brain and nervous system. So, in this section, we'll focus on the primary ways of regulating the nervous system to reduce symptoms of depression, anxiety, and stress.

Building or enhancing brain health is for everyone, and these are techniques that you can put into place immediately. In our experience, the majority of women prefer strategies that they can do on their own, because it makes them feel in control of their own mental health while still having access to a safety net when needed.

The Tools for Building Brain Health

I want to introduce you to two kinds of tools that were first introduced by Dr. Bessel van der Kolk.[1] The first are bottom-up tools, and they are designed to directly regulate the brain and autonomic nervous system (our automatic responses). Thinking back to the Autonomic Ladder, bottom-up strategies are the tools that we can use to move us from the sympathetic state (middle of ladder) or the dorsal vagal state (bottom of ladder) back up the ladder to our neurobiologically calm ventral vagal state (top of ladder). For depression, anxiety, and stress, these are first-line strategies—primary go-to tools that build neuroplasticity—and every time you use them, you are building brain health.

Top-down tools are those that work by focusing on the higher, thinking centres of our brain (e.g., cognitive behaviour therapy). They can't directly regulate the brain and nervous system because they work on a different part of the brain—the logical, thinking parts. They are useful as second-line strategies—after your brain and nervous system are regulated—and they may help to maintain you in a regulated state.

The first step in managing your own brain health is to know where you're at by working through some self-assessments to get a good sense of the kind and level of your symptoms. Your symptoms are the language of dysregulation. If you are experiencing mild symptoms, your brain and nervous system are mildly dysregulated. If you have moderate or severe symptoms, your brain and nervous system are more dysregulated.

Regardless of where you're at, start by implementing bottom-up strategies regularly in your day, as they are the foundation of brain health. Experiment with the top-down strategies (one or two at a time, maximum) to see if they have additional brain health benefits for you.

As with all behaviour changes, small steps bring success. Create a daily plan. What I recommend to my clients is that they practice their brain-based tools just before they eat a meal. Attaching a new habit to something that is already part of your life (like supper) acts as a reminder to do it. Finally, when you are working on a new habit, it can be helpful to journal or keep notes on your success and struggles.

Bottom-Up Strategies

Regulating Your Nervous System

Below are three bottom-up, brain-based strategies that I recommend you implement daily and any time that you feel that you are moving from a place of ventral vagal safety down the ladder to the sympathetic or dorsal vagal states. Our team fondly calls this package the BEE Protocol, which stands for Breathing, Ears, and Eyes, and we recommend you follow them in order of steps 1, 2, and then 3. Altogether, the BEE Protocol can take as little as five minutes.

Step 1: Deep Breathing Deep breathing is a physiological reset of sorts—when you breathe deeply, the pressure in your abdomen presses on your vagal nerve, signalling to your brain that you are safe.[2] In effect, it helps your body interrupt its natural, protective response to fear and threat, with physiological outcomes such as lowered blood pressure.

You can practice deep breathing any time, anywhere—on the train, lying in bed, sitting at your office desk, at your kitchen table.

Here is the routine: Close your eyes, relax your shoulders, and put your hand on your belly. Breathe in slowly and fully through your nose until you feel your abdomen pressing against your spine. Hold for a count of 4. Then slowly release your breath out through your mouth for a count of 6. Repeat this process for 1 to 5 minutes. You can also put your hand over your heart during this exercise, as in the Hand on Heart exercise mentioned earlier.

Step 2: Ear Exercise The vagus nerve travels very close to your inner ear, and so we can access it to stimulate it through our ears. The principle is the same as deep breathing: this exercise applies pressure to each branch of the vagus nerve, sending the signal to your brain that you are safe, and your nervous system can stand down. For this exercise, begin with one ear. If you are starting with your left ear, place your left index finger above the cartilage shelf in your ear (the small ridge you feel just above your ear canal) and make small circles, moving your finger in a clockwise direction for twenty times. Then, repeat with your right ear, using your right index finger.

Step 3: The Basic Exercise (Eyes)[3] This exercise also calms your vagus nerve by realigning your cervical vertebrae and enhancing blood flow to the brainstem, helping your vagus nerve to function better.[4] You can do it sitting up or lying on your back (knees bent for comfort).

1. Interlock your fingers and place your hands behind your neck with your thumbs resting on your neck.
2. Begin in the neutral position of looking straight ahead. Don't move your head—it stays in this position.
3. Look toward one elbow, just moving your eyes. Hold that

position for one minute, or until you feel the urge to sigh, yawn, or take a deep breath.

4. Come back to the neutral position, with your eyes looking straight ahead, and rest.

5. When you are ready, look toward your other elbow, again just moving your eyes. Hold this position for one minute, or until you feel the urge to sigh, yawn, or take a deep breath. That's it!

You can do the Basic Exercise daily or a few times a week. It's a good exercise both for keeping your nervous system tuned up and for re-regulating your nervous system if you have slid down the ladder.

Emotional Freedom Technique (EFT) The emotional freedom technique was originally designed for treating post-traumatic stress disorder, but well over one hundred studies show that it is effective and fast at lowering depression, anxiety, and stress symptoms and physiological measures.[5, 6, 7] EFT uses a systematic process of tapping along the facial, chest, and hand meridian points while listening to an affirming script. In a recently published study, researchers found that the depression and anxiety scores of pregnant women who practiced EFT regularly until six months postpartum were lowered 30 percent and 23 percent respectively, moving them out of the range of clinical depression and anxiety.[8] There are several excellent YouTube videos demonstrating EFT, especially those by social worker Julie Schiffman.

Listening to Music[9] Listening to music is an easy, effective way of regulating your vagal nervous system to reduce symptoms of depression, anxiety, and stress. Music creates sound vibrations that travel into our ears and vibrate our eardrums. Because the vagus nerve runs very close to our eardrum, anything that causes the eardrum to vibrate physically activates the vagus nerve, too, triggering the calming, parasympathetic nervous system.[10] Recent investigations are also exploring the effect of *specific* vibrations that have an especially powerful effect on slowing our heart rate breathing, decreasing blood pressure, and reducing anxiety and stress.[11] Overall, resources recommend listening (through headphones) to calming harp music within the frequencies of 174 Hz, 417 Hz, 444 Hz, 528 Hz, or 639 Hz, or calming Mozart effect music for thirty minutes per day.[12]

Singing If you enjoy singing, then regulating your vagus nerve this way will be a natural and easy strategy for you. The vagus nerve runs close to, and controls, the pharynx and larynx at the back of your throat. When you sing loudly, hum, or chant, you activate the vagal nerve. Interestingly, a recent study showed that 73 percent of new mothers who participated in an online singing intervention reduced their symptoms of postpartum depression, anxiety, and stress and increased their sense of life satisfaction and worthwhileness.[13] The investigators also noted that singing is associated with social bonding, relaxation, and social support. Although the researchers didn't investigate the neurobiological reasons for the positive effects of the group singing, all reflect a re-regulated nervous system. And finally, perhaps less pleasant than singing, loud gargling for ten seconds activates the vagus nerve in the same way as loud singing.

Mindfulness If you find that the changes of pregnancy and new motherhood feel daunting, mindfulness may help. Change of any sort involves first knowing and noticing where we're at, settling our bodies, and redirecting our unhealthy thoughts, feelings, and actions to healthy ones. Mindfulness is a strategy that helps you to be aware of your body responses, thoughts, and emotions so that you can use them to make purposeful decisions about what to put your attention on.[14] Think of mindfulness as stepping off a treadmill and giving yourself the opportunity to pause, slow down, and to take charge again of your thoughts, emotions, and actions. The goal is to learn to focus on things that build you up—not deflate you and tear you down—and this is why it works well for lessening the symptoms of depression and anxiety.

I've included mindfulness in the bottom-up section because it is a very helpful practice for training you to listen to your body. It's been used as a mainstay treatment in cancer care for years because its overall effects on the body are so recuperative.[15] And as I've shared earlier, our neuro-dysregulation is always detected first in the body—that gut twinge, the tension that creeps into our neck and shoulders, our all-day fatigue. When you learn to read your body's dysregulation as a beneficial sign that all is not well, then you can implement tools to re-set it.

One of the consequences of an overwhelming life experience (as a child or adult) is that we may disconnect from our body. At first, when I studied the neurobiology of depression, anxiety, and stress, I hadn't a clue what that meant. But when I spent time firsthand in brain-based grief counselling after my mother passed away, Dr. Elizabeth Atwell taught me how to regulate my brain and nervous system. In a session, she would typically begin by asking, "What do you notice in your body?" and I would respond, "I have no idea." I wasn't used to turning my attention to my fatigue or pain. Many women whom I have counselled have been in the same place. Most had grown up in a family where everyone else's needs took precedence, and they perfected the strategy of shoving their needs (and desires) down deep. And while that strategy can serve us well for a time, it collapses at some point, manifesting as depression, anxiety, stress, grief and loss, frustration, or anger—or all of the above.

To make mindfulness a habit, pick a point in your day (for instance, when you are in the shower or eating your lunch) and focus on what you are doing. If you are in the shower, notice the smell, the temperature and feel of the water, the sight of the glistening water drops, the feeling of the water on your arms. When your thoughts escape the shower and wander away toward what's for dinner, for example, just bring them back to the shower. With practice, you'll develop a habit of diverting your attention from distractions that waste your time and emotional energy to helpful, healthful thoughts and activities. If you need help getting started, there are many free apps that provide guided mindful-based tools. Dr. Deb Dana has several useful meditative mindfulness recordings that are specifically designed to be practiced as part of a brain-based protocol.[16]

Top-Down Strategies

Cultivate Trusted Relationships Cultivating trusted relationships is a requisite strategy for everyone, regardless of how social you judge yourself to be. I've shared how safe relationships protect you from depression, anxiety, and stress, but they can also lessen the intensity of your symptoms. A recent review showed that supportive relationships enhance pregnant women's positive emotions; increase their quality of life, sense of worth, confidence, and trust; and help them to feel more connected to their partner.[17] Harkening back to the neurobiology of relationships, these are features that make us feel inherently safe.

The problem with depression, anxiety, and stress is that they often drive women to connect *less* at a time when they need to connect *more*. One of the consequences of neural dysregulation is that we withdraw from others. When we've reached out for help, and help hasn't come (e.g., our needs have been dismissed or ignored), then our brain and nervous system move into a freeze state (bottom of ladder model) where we find greater safety in detachment. We may also withdraw from others because we feel shame about where we're at, embarrassed about our current state or that we need help, or are simply too drained and exhausted to expend the effort to reach out.

But the evidence for social support decreasing symptoms of depression, anxiety, and stress is strong.[18] Having good support not only soothes our emotions, makes us feel heard and understood, and gives us alternate perspectives but it also reduces our levels of stress hormones that keep us in a keyed-up state. Rather than detaching from your most trusted supports, connect with them. For many women I've counselled, this is a huge step, but when they take it, they find that the comfort and help they receive is well worth the vulnerability they feel. Reaching out might be to simply sit together, for them to have minimal expectations of you, to chat over coffee, or to go for a silent walk together and just appreciate the co-regulating presence of a trusted companion.

Other women I've served in counselling have felt they haven't had a voice. They've been in relationships as children or adults where they couldn't express their needs because it came with criticism, unpredictable backlash, anger, repeated disappointment at being dismissed, and woundedness at being not seen or heard—anything but safety. Over time, they learned to squash their needs to the point where they couldn't even identify them. Neurobiologically, many of them would place themselves at the bottom rung of the ladder model because they felt shut down so much of the time. As you can, practice saying what you need from trusted friends and family. You might say, "What I need right now is . . ." or "What would make me feel better in this moment is . . ." or "It would help me most if . . ."

To end this section, I want to return to the notion of neurobiological safety. Dr. Dan Siegel, a Harvard University–trained psychiatrist and clinical professor of psychiatry at UCLA School of Medicine, is renowned for his work on the biology of relationships. His work has shifted our whole idea of relationships, showing that when partners experience conflict and arguments, it doesn't just produce anger, irritability, and frustration. It goes much deeper to impact each person's nervous system, rewiring the brain and the nervous system in real time, including the unborn baby.[19, 20, 21]

Nature Spending time in nature is an easy and powerful way of restoring a sense of peace and groundedness when we are triggered by life challenges. Nature therapy not only delights our senses but also induces mental and physiological relaxation. It reduces our stress hormones, lowers our heart rate variability (a sign of neural regulation!), improves our blood sugar levels, strengthens our immune system so that we can fight infection better, and increases our parasympathetic nervous system activity, which is our body's calm, regulated state. Natural settings enable us to recover from stress faster and give us the comforting sense that there is a higher purpose—something "greater than oneself." For me, being in nature has always been foundational to my brain health. Indeed, it was a major reason why, in our late fifties, my husband and I moved with our son to a small farm and now raise sheep. Our sheep give me an immense sense of peace, calm, and pleasure.

Being in nature also replenishes our brain's ability to focus and put our attention on the important—a phenomenon called directed attention—which brings rest, restoration, and relaxation. And studies have found that even just spending time in small green spaces—such as being in your garden or populating your living and working spaces with plants and wood furniture—reduces depression, anxiety, and stress.

Making daily time in nature a habit while you're pregnant not only helps to reduce symptoms of depression, anxiety, and stress, but it is also something you can carry forward after your baby is born. Walking with your infant, toddler, or preschooler in nature helps your child regulate their emotions; develop their curiosity, creativity, attention, and intellect; strengthen their socio-emotional development; and build your relationship attachment as you spend time in undistracted interaction. Ask yourself: How much time do I spend in nature? Could I commit to fifteen or thirty minutes each day?

Sleep Hygiene If you are not feeling rested when you wake up in the morning, improving your sleep can make an immediate improvement in your mental health. Not only is poor sleep a risk factor for depression, anxiety, and stress, but it also tends to keep your symptoms elevated and harder to manage. The National Sleep Foundation recommends seven to nine hours' sleep per night, but by the third trimester, three-quarters of pregnant women experience interrupted sleep cycles due to waking nightly to reposition themselves or go to the bathroom. Overall, judge your sleep quality by how refreshed you feel when you awake.

Some strategies for establishing good sleep hygiene are:

- creating a relaxing bedtime routine, such as having a bath or reading
- going to bed and getting up at the same time each day
- limiting caffeinated drinks
- sleeping on your side with a pillow under your belly or between your knees

- using a weighted blanket
- eliminating electronics at least one hour before bedtime
- exercising during the day
- practicing progressive relaxation or hand-on-heart strategies once in bed
- taking a sleep assessment (if you snore)
- napping during the day (if this doesn't keep you up all night)

Symptom Tracking When you are experiencing symptoms of depression, anxiety, and/or stress, it's helpful to monitor your level of distress on a regular basis. On its own, symptom tracking doesn't act to lessen depression, anxiety, or stress symptoms. Its role is to help you to track your level of symptoms so that you know which tools are helping and which are not so that you can pivot early to a new strategy. You can use the same assessments in earlier chapters to track your levels of symptoms any time you want to check in on yourself. There are also several free mood tracking apps available.

Spiritual Practices If you're struggling with the transition of pregnancy, studies show that spiritual practices can help. Some studies have described a growing interest in spiritual practices, such as meditation, thanksgiving/gratitude, and prayer, in helping pregnant women adjust in the midst of significant transition.[22] For instance, in a study of almost 18,000 women in Sweden who were surveyed during the COVID-19 pandemic, 41 percent indicated that they took some moments to pray (have inner dialogue addressed to God or something greater than themselves) and/or meditate, and most (75 percent) reflected on the meaning and purpose of life altering as they transitioned to motherhood. For some, spiritual practices help to ground them emotionally, while for others they are part of making meaning and rethinking their purpose in life. There is some evidence that prayer also has an impact on the vagus nerve, likely because it induces a sense of safety and well-being.[23] If you have never adopted spiritual practices but would like to start, there are even pregnancy prayer apps!

Exercise We all know the importance of exercise for our physical health, and it has many added benefits for pregnant women, such as reducing lower back and pelvic pain and the risk of gestational hypertension. It's also effective at preventing and treating mental health problems, in part because it addresses some of the physiological elements, such as inflammation and immune function.[24, 25] Research shows that all kinds of exercise—walking, stationary bicycling, stretching, yoga, and relaxation—help reduce symptoms of depression, anxiety, and stress by as much as 50 percent and increase the speed of recovery by 50 percent. In one study, 82 percent of pregnant women who exercised lowered their depression symptoms compared to 26 percent of women who didn't. Another review of trials of physical exercise and prenatal depression concluded that physical activity as little as one to three times per week significantly reduces depression symptoms in pregnant women.

And exercise is safe for pregnant women who don't have obstetric or medical complications. The American College of Obstetricians and Gynecologists (ACOG) recommends thirty to sixty minutes of moderate intensity aerobic exercise—walking, stationary cycling, dancing, resistance exercises, stretching, or water aerobics—during pregnancy and the postpartum period, three to four times per week. However, if you have been sedentary prior to pregnancy, begin exercising gradually, working up to a moderate level of intensity. If you have any sort of obstetric or medical complications (e.g., high blood pressure, placenta previa, cardiovascular disease, anemia, multiple gestation), don't start an exercise program without checking in with your prenatal care provider first.

An additional bottom-up, neurological benefit of exercise that I find fascinating is that it provides opportunity for the nervous system to make shifts between a calm, relaxed bodily state (during rest) and an activated state (during exercise).[26] When we exercise, our sympathetic nervous system is naturally stimulated to increase our heart rate and respiratory rate, direct extra blood to our muscles, etc., as we run, dance, stretch, or perform weight training. A healthy nervous system makes an efficient switch between calm and activation, and back to calm again. It's a bit like learning to drive a standard vehicle. You want your gear shifts to be as smooth and effortless as possible! Finally, exercise (lifting weights and aerobic) has been shown to stimulate the vagus nerve, which may in part explain its beneficial effects on depression, anxiety, and stress.[27]

Progressive Muscle Relaxation If you are experiencing tension as part of your symptoms of depression, anxiety, or stress, progressive muscle relaxation can help. Progressive muscle relaxation involves tensing and relaxing your muscles, systematically moving through all the major muscle groups in your body. Studies show that muscle relaxation can reduce symptoms of depression, anxiety, and stress by as much as 50 percent, especially when combined with other strategies such as CBT. Recent trials in pregnant women have also shown that combining progressive relaxation with guided imagery (visualization of peaceful settings) reduces stress and anxiety scores on assessments, lowers heart rate, decreases levels of stress chemicals that are released into our blood when we experience stress, and induces a sense of calm.[28] In other words, this simple tool can shift not only your mood but your physiological parameters as well!

To get you started, I've outlined an exercise that you can

implement right now. For the first week or two, try this exercise twice a day.

1. Find a quiet setting where you can be undisturbed for about fifteen minutes.
2. Begin by sitting in a comfortable position, closing your eyes, and letting your body relax or go loose. Take five slow, deep breaths.
3. Then, begin with a certain part of your body, such as your feet, and curl your toes for five seconds, focusing on your toes and taking slow, deep breaths.
4. Next, quickly relax your tensed toes, exhaling as you release the muscles. The goal is to notice the difference between the tension and relaxed feeling. Stay relaxed for about fifteen seconds, and then move on to another muscle group and repeat for the remaining minutes.
5. Over the fifteen minutes, you don't have to get through all muscle groups, though you may want to work up your body, tensing and relaxing your lower leg and foot (move your toes toward you), leg (squeeze your thigh muscles), hands (squeeze into fists), arm (tighten your biceps by drawing your forearm—and clenched fist—toward your shoulder to make a muscle), buttocks (tighten and pull together), stomach (suck in), chest (tighten by taking a deep breath), neck and shoulders (raise to touch ears), mouth (open wide), eyes (shut tightly), and forehead (raise eyebrows up). Try tensing and relaxing both sides of your body.

The goal of progressive relaxation is to reduce muscle tension, putting you in a relaxed, calm state. It will also enhance your body awareness as you compare and contrast what it feels like to tense and relax muscles. If you've struggled with anxiety- or stress-related tension for a long time, it's likely that you've experienced muscular tension so persistently that you may not know what physical relaxation feels like.

Self-Managed Counselling I define self-managed counselling as any online- or workbook-based counselling that you work through on your own. If you want a strategy that provides a broad base of education and information about depression, anxiety, and stress as well as techniques to address them, this may be helpful. Good sources can teach us a lot about what's going on in our brain and body. As with all top-down strategies, my advice is that they are used as an adjunct to brain-based work—both of which you can do on your own if you choose.

At times, I have recommended workbooks or online courses to pregnant women that I have counselled. Typically, we would do brain-based work in their session, and then I would assign a chapter or module to work through before our next visit. We would debrief about their homework, and I would answer any questions they have. Some of the online courses and workbooks I have used in this capacity are: our HOPE Platform;[29] *The Resilience Workbook* (Glenn R. Schiraldi); *The Cognitive Behavioral Workbook for Depression*, second edition (William J. Knaus); and *The Set Boundaries Workbook* (Nedra Glover Tawwab).

Professional Support

If you have tried several self-management strategies and are finding that you need additional support, or your symptoms are at a severe level, professional support might be a consideration. In this book,

I have honoured the preference for many women to manage their brain health on their own. At the same time, when we have severe symptoms or experience significantly distressing situations in our lives, it can be helpful to move through the early, acute distress with a supportive professional. This is especially true when the situation involves the partner as well and the immensity of the circumstance makes it difficult to lean on each other for support.

Here is a five-question self-assessment that you can use to decide whether getting professional support is a good next step for you. For each question, identify the degree to which the statement is like you.

CHECKING IN

Is It Time to Get Help?

STATEMENT	This is exactly like me.	This is somewhat like me.	This isn't like me at all.
I feel like I'm in the same place as I was a month ago.			
I've tried several things on my own, but I don't feel like they're enough.			
I feel worse than I did a month ago.			
I would value the chance to talk to someone about my problems.			
I don't have the energy or motivation to keep working at things on my own.			

If you answered most of the questions with "This is exactly like me" or "This is somewhat like me," then it's a good time to think about engaging some professional support. Because many women put others' needs before their own, I encourage you to consider therapy a gift to yourself, much like you might think of a spa day as a treat.

In the next part of the chapter, I'll walk you through how to navigate the world of therapy if this is new to you. The most important consideration when it comes to therapy is the therapist. With the right practitioner, your growth can be expedited. But finding that person can be a bit like dating—it has to be a good match for it to work. Many counsellors offer a fifteen-minute pre-session before you sign an agreement to determine whether you and the counsellor will work well together. Your goal in that pre-session is to focus on the fit, noticing whether you connect with the counsellor right away, the degree of ease and comfort you feel with them, and whether their approach sounds like it fits your tendencies and preferences. If it becomes clear in the introductory meeting that the match between you and the counsellor isn't what you had hoped for, simply thank them for their time. They want the best for you, too, and an ineffective fit simply delays your healing.

You'll know that you've got the best therapist *for you* when:

- you feel comfortable and at ease to talk about sensitive topics
- you sense the therapist is understanding and empathic, and respects you and your wishes
- you feel heard and listened to
- the therapist helps you to make sense of your confusion (i.e., brings clarity)
- you can cry, and the therapist is a comforting presence

- although the therapist may not have gone through the exact same experience as you have, you feel that they understand the emotions and challenges of the experience
- you are changing in the direction you want to go, meeting the goals you want to attain, and learning more about yourself along the journey

There are many kinds of arrangements, and you can work with a therapist to determine what is best for you and what you are going through. In my practice, I serve some women regularly (e.g., every week or two) and others periodically (e.g., every few months for a few sessions) for those who want support with specific life situations that have come up or for a brain-nervous system tune-up. From a delivery standpoint, you can choose a practitioner who offers therapy face-to-face, online, or both. Even brain-based therapies can be offered online. Most important, as you solidify your arrangement, you remain in control of your mental health. You choose the timing and work with your practitioner to decide on the best course of action. You can start with one kind of therapy, and if it isn't a good fit for you, then you can move on to a different sort. Being informed about the options and knowing yourself and your preferences is a good starting place.

When you meet a therapist for the first time, ask what approach they use (there are several different approaches to counselling) and see whether it sounds like a good fit for you. You don't have to know all the possible approaches. The therapist's job is to explain their approach in a way that helps you to understand whether it's a good fit for you or not. Most therapists use several kinds of therapy, so if one doesn't work, you can agree to switch to another. Broadly, therapies are divided into brain-based or talking therapies.

Brain-Based Therapies

For depression, anxiety, stress, and trauma (adult or early childhood), my best advice is to look for someone who uses research-supported, brain-based therapies because they offer the fastest, most complete, most effective approaches to directly regulating the nervous system and reducing distress.[30] In addition, brain-based techniques support neuroplasticity so that the work you do with the therapist has lasting effects—and you'll learn how to keep your brain and nervous system tuned up. I use brain-based therapies with all my clients because we all need to learn and practice brain care as we face dysregulating life situations on a daily basis.

Five of the most widely used brain-based therapies are:

- *Neurofeedback:* a therapy that helps identify unhealthy dysregulated brain wave patterns and to help the brain recover, and therefore is helpful for insomnia, trauma, depression, anxiety, and stress.
- *Eye Movement Desensitization and Reprocessing (EMDR):* a therapy that helps to completely process life experiences that continue to affect you, reducing symptoms of depression, anxiety, grief, and loss, eating disorders, panic attacks, and chronic illness.[31, 32, 33]
- *Brainspotting:* a therapy developed by Dr. David Grand that helps with accessing unprocessed life experiences in the subcortical brain by using points in your field of vision, reducing depression, anxiety, grief, and loss, phobias, and panic attacks, and improving elite performance.[34, 35]
- *Safe and Sound Protocol:* a therapy developed by Dr. Stephen Porges that restores balance to the nervous system by

teaching it to feel safe; reducing depression, anxiety, and stress symptoms; and improving confidence, fear, poor emotional control, trust, and social engagement.

- *Tomatis Therapy:* a therapy developed by Dr. Alfred Tomatis that uses music to stimulate the ear and nervous system to promote brain health through neuroplasticity and vagus nerve regulation.[36, 37]

Talk Therapies

Talk therapies may be valuable adjuncts to brain-based approaches. In my practice, I use brain-based techniques as the core therapy, and then I might bring in the principles of other therapies to teach my clients, for example, how to implement new habits, set boundaries, or change relationship patterns that have been established as a consequence of trauma wounds.

Cognitive Behaviour Therapy

If you are struggling with repetitive, distressing thoughts, then cognitive behaviour therapy (CBT) might be helpful. Many counsellors use cognitive behaviour therapy to help pregnant women reduce their symptoms of depression, anxiety, and stress, but you can practice its principles on your own as well.

CBT is one of the most widely researched and practiced therapies. But research shows its effectiveness in the perinatal period is moderate at best, and the effects are not long-lasting, with 19 percent to 47 percent of people relapsing to a pre-therapy level of symptoms within a few months.[38, 39, 40, 41]

CBT's strategies are based on the core idea that your beliefs, thoughts, emotions, and body sensations are interconnected so that, for instance, your beliefs drive your thoughts, which affect your emotions, and then you respond with some sort of behaviour. For example, if you believe that other couples in your prenatal class have it all together, you might be consumed with unhealthy, comparative thoughts during the class (e.g., "She looks great: way better than me," "They look so happy; I bet they never fight like we do") that prevent you from hearing what the prenatal instructor is teaching. Feelings of doubt and insecurity follow, and before you know it, you avoid socializing with other women during the break and stop participating in class—experiences that otherwise might have been helpful to you (and others!). The goal of cognitive behaviour therapy is to change your thinking to be more realistic (e.g., "She doesn't look better than me. We all look different than we're used to") and the notion is that healthier thinking reduces symptoms of depression, anxiety, and stress, so that you can act differently.

But new neuroscience has challenged researchers' and clinicians' views of the usefulness of traditional CBT. A significant challenge of CBT is that when we experience depression, anxiety, or stress, our prefrontal, thinking parts of our brain can't exert control over the parts of our brain that are reacting to threat.[42] It is like asking our higher thinking centres to do something they were not meant to do. Ultimately, the process of changing an unhealthy thought happens in the prefrontal cortex and doesn't directly target the parts of our brain and nervous system that are activated by threat. Thus, we are required to put in effort to identify and reformulate a thought while our brain and nervous system are in an activated state—a feat that is almost impossible.[43]

Is there a place for developing awareness of your thoughts, recognizing unhealthy thought patterns, and taking control of your repetitive thinking? Absolutely! I place CBT strategies in a bucket of top-down tools that enhance your awareness of your body's reactions, thoughts, and emotions that you experience in triggering situations; then, with the recognition that your brain and nervous system are dysregulated, you can implement brain-based tools to re-regulate your system. Put another way, while traditional CBT prioritizes building awareness so you can swap unhealthy for healthy thoughts, new neuroscience views this triggering of body responses, thoughts, and feelings as signs that your brain and nervous system are dysregulated.

If you like, you can track your responses to triggering situations in the CBT-based tool, the Thought Record, that follows.

THE THOUGHT RECORD[44]

Situation
What happened? Where were you? Who was with you?

Feeling/Emotion
What did you feel? Rate the strength of the emotion from 0 percent to 100 percent.

Negative Automatic Thought
What thoughts or images went through your mind?

Evidence for Negative Thought
What evidence supports your negative thought?

Evidence Against Negative Thought
What evidence doesn't support your negative thought?

Alternative, Realistic, Balanced Thought
Looking at all the evidence, what is a different, more realistic, and balanced thought?

New Feeling/Emotion
How do you feel when you consider that thought?

CBT has clarified the kinds of unhelpful thought patterns we experience, which I think are quite helpful to understand as triggering thoughts. These include:

- All-or-nothing thinking: you see things in black and white ("If I can't manage my life when I'm pregnant, I'll be a terrible mother").
- Overgeneralization: you draw conclusions about who you are and your abilities from one single incident versus a realistic assessment from a number of situations ("I didn't know the answer to that question in prenatal classes. I'm stupid").
- Selective filtering: you focus on the negative parts of a conversation or situation and ignore the other aspects. For example, you replay a relative's comment about how much you've "blossomed" since she last saw you and ignore or forget all the comments she made about how healthy you looked, how nice your house was, and how happy you and your partner seemed.
- Magnification: you blow a situation out of proportion or imagine the worst possible outcome ("I gained two pounds this week! I'm harming the baby!").
- Personalization: you personalize an external event when in reality there isn't a connection. For example, your boss doesn't make eye contact with you as she walks past you in the hall, and you interpret that to mean that you have done something wrong, or your work is sub-standard.
- Labeling, where you tell yourself, "I am a [label]." For example, your partner made a comment about how big you are getting (partners, don't do this!), and you said to yourself, "I am ugly!"

- *Should*s and *must*s: you think or say, "I should" or "I shouldn't," creating unrealistic expectations for yourself. ("When the baby is born, I should join a baby swimming class, a baby library program, a weight-loss program, a mother-baby walking group, and a new mothers' coffee group.")

From a neuroscience perspective, these automatic, triggering thought patterns are generally built during childhood amid circumstances that felt unsafe. They tend to be subtle whispers that sound like our own voice and so we don't even notice them. When you identify these thoughts or their effects on you (tension, stomach knots, headache, stress, and anxiety), practice your bottom-up, brain-based tools.

Acceptance and Commitment Therapy

If you struggle with accepting challenging life circumstances, then acceptance and commitment therapy (ACT) might be a good fit for you. And while there are trained ACT therapists, you can also implement the principles in your life on your own.

Think of acceptance as the opposite of resistance and avoidance, which is often our default strategy when we're faced with a difficult situation and emotions. What does resistance and avoidance look like? It's physical tension (tense, raised shoulders, clenched jaw, and knot-in-stomach syndrome, tensed forehead), and repetitive, ruminative thoughts (replaying the situation or distressing thoughts over and over). It's also being emotionally stuck in high stress, anxiety, or depression.

Acceptance feels counterintuitive, like you are giving up your goals or passively remaining in difficult situations—but it's the opposite. It's accepting your situation, thoughts, and feelings, allowing the realities of the good and bad to exist together side by side instead of letting your emotional energy be consumed by an internal battle. I know that sounds strange, but it's far healthier. Research shows that acceptance results in less psychological distress, so you have the capacity to move toward the goals that are important to you and consistent with your values. Try this exercise: Think about a situation or problem that creates distress for you and instead of shoving it down below the surface or ignoring it, ask, "Why am I having this thought or feeling?" and "What is this telling me about myself at this moment?" Then think about simply accepting the situation. What happens to your emotions? Your body? When I do this, my mind feels soothed, my forehead relaxes, my shoulders drop, and I feel myself breathe easily. It feels . . . easier.

From a brain-body perspective, I suggest that when we are in resistance, we are in the fight-or-flight place on the ladder model. We're fighting against our situation (and often ourselves), and our body is supporting us by gearing up with muscle tension and other responses. But the soothing calm you feel when you accept a situation is a reflection of being in the upper part of the ladder, the ventral vagal place, where your brain can be creative, and you can discover solutions.

Medication

At this point, you might be wondering about whether medication is an option during pregnancy. Several studies have found that therapy is as effective as taking medication, such as antidepressants, for the majority of women with sub-clinical, mild, and moderate symptoms of depression and anxiety. For this reason, therapy is recommended as the main form of treatment for pregnant women.

However, sometimes when our symptoms are so overwhelming that we have trouble carrying on with our daily lives, medication can provide significant relief—and antidepressants can be prescribed for both depression and anxiety. Pregnant women with *severe* symptoms who may not have the energy, motivation, or ability to concentrate to get better from therapy alone benefit the most from a combination of therapy and an antidepressant. Research shows that medication is more effective and faster acting with therapy, and they should be combined for the best results; for this reason, medication alone is not recommended. From a practical standpoint, women starting on medication are often quite distressed and therefore medication is typically started first with therapy added a few weeks or months later when the antidepressant has started to work.

Deciding whether or not to take an antidepressant during pregnancy is a process filled with angst for 2 out of 3 women.[45] One of the realities of antidepressants is that only half of pregnant women with moderate to severe depression experience relief, and finding an effective antidepressant can take several cycles of starting on one, increasing the dosage, experiencing side effects and worsening mood, decreasing the dosage, weaning off, and starting on the next one. You know an antidepressant is a good fit for you when it improves your mood symptoms, your appetite is good, you sleep better, you have more energy, and you enjoy life again.

The first-line antidepressants for women with moderate to severe symptoms of depression or anxiety in pregnancy is a class of medications called selective serotonin reuptake inhibitors (SSRIs) such as sertraline (Zoloft) or citalopram (Celexa). Zoloft and Celexa are recommended because there is little transfer in utero and in breastmilk, and they have few side effects. It can take a few weeks to start to feel better, with noticeable results by four to six weeks.

If an SSRI isn't effective for you, your doctor may prescribe another type of medication that has proven safety in pregnancy, such as a serotonin and norepinephrine reuptake inhibitor (SNRI) like duloxetine (Cymbalta) or venlafaxine (Effexor); an antidepressant like bupropion (Wellbutrin); or a tricyclic antidepressant (TCA) like nortriptyline (Pamelor) or desipramine (Norpramin). Some women experience side effects, such as stomach upset (e.g., diarrhea, nausea, decreased appetite), headache, dreams, dry mouth, jitteriness or agitation, insomnia, and sexual effects (e.g., decreased libido). If the medication is a good fit for you, the side effects are generally only felt for the first two weeks after starting the medication and improve after that. I'll discuss medication in more detail in the next chapter.

The brain health strategies in this chapter are simple but highly effective tools that put you in charge of your mental health. My hope is that they help you to feel confident and empowered to optimize you and your baby's mental health.

CHAPTER 8

Is Medication a Good Choice for You?

When women think of taking medications in pregnancy, they often think of the thalidomide scare of the 1950s and 1960s where infants of women who took thalidomide for pregnancy nausea and vomiting suffered major congenital anomalies. In that era, doctors and researchers didn't understand that medications could cross the placenta. No research tested thalidomide during pregnancy, and it was five years before the connection between the drug and infant deformities was made. Today, medications for use in pregnancy are tested extensively. At this point, we don't see evidence that current antidepressants that are recommended during pregnancy are linked to birth defects.

New US-based data show that antidepressant use is on the rise, having increased steadily over the past twenty years in both men and women. And this usage parallels the rise of mental health problems we see globally. However, about twice as many women outside of pregnancy take antidepressants (19 percent) as men (10 percent),[1] making the issue of antidepressants an important one for planning pregnancy. In fact, half of women who experience depression or anxiety say that it shapes their family planning decisions, including the timing (they want to be emotionally well before getting pregnant), concern for relapse, and indecision about the type of treatment they should choose.

Half of women that I counsel and who are trying to get pregnant within a year say that they plan to stay on antidepressants through their pregnancy, and my experience is reflected in current research.[2] A recent study of more than 57,000 pregnant women showed that more than 50 percent come off their antidepressants without any other supports in place.[3] A 50–50 split like this tells me that: (1) the decision is hard, and (2) there isn't one answer that is right for everyone. Women who have found good symptom control with an antidepressant are more inclined to continue with it throughout pregnancy. And staying on your antidepressant can be reassuring—many women feel secure and stable on their dosage and type of antidepressant, and, for some, it took a lot of adjustments (and feeling crappy) to get there. However, you may still require a change in the kind of antidepressant if the one you're on isn't recommended in pregnancy. The safest strategy is to discuss your antidepressant therapy with your physician or psychiatrist before you get pregnant. That way, if you need to change antidepressants because the one you are taking isn't safe for pregnancy, you have time to wean off and start another. If you and your physician agree that you could stop your medication, you have time to gradually stop it and connect in with other supports as necessary.

In every chapter, I've discussed topics within the neuroscience of perinatal mental health because I firmly believe that this is the direction we must go if we are to support pregnant women and their babies optimally. Antidepressants by their very nature regulate the brain and nervous system. They are designed to bring brain chemicals within an ideal range, thereby lessening symptoms. The "bottom-up" tools in this book are the non-medication versions of how to regulate the brain and nervous system and foster neuroplasticity. Am I saying medications are bad or unnecessary? No. But I am suggesting that we now have effective and easy approaches to improving brain health that offer competitive alternatives to medication.

This chapter is for you if you are wondering about whether you should go on—or off—medications as you consider or plan a pregnancy, are pregnant now, or are thinking about medications as you head into new motherhood. Two out of three women facing decisions about going on or off antidepressants experience a lot of conflict and stress about the decision.[4] One of the main problems that women experience is confusion about the different stories and opinions circulating about pregnancy and antidepressants so that it's hard to know what information is reliable. In this chapter, you'll find our most up-to-date evidence to guide your decisions on the benefits and downsides of medications at each of these critical points, questions to consider in making your decision, how to have medication-related discussions with your doctor, and how your partner can be involved in this decision process.

What to Know About Taking Medication *Before* Pregnancy

If you're wondering about whether to stop medication before you become pregnant, one key thing to consider is your medical history. Most women with moderate to severe depression or anxiety symptoms have also experienced one or more episodes of depression or persistent, high anxiety in the past, and this makes them more likely to relapse if they stop taking their antidepressant. Which is why many experts recommend that women who were on antidepressants before pregnancy for moderate to severe depression, anxiety, or a combination continue to use them throughout the pregnancy and after delivery.

Certain antidepressants, such as SSRIs, are better suited for pregnancy and postpartum because they have fewer side effects for you and your baby, so if you are planning a pregnancy, you should talk to your doctor about the specific medication you are taking. For example, one SSRI, paroxetine (Paxil), carries a small risk— 0.2 percent to 0.4 percent—of heart malformations for the baby, and you and your doctor may decide that another SSRI is a better option.[5] If a change is needed, your doctor will help you make that transition, which will involve decreasing the dose of your current medication and gradually increasing the new one. This can be unsettling, especially if a certain one has been working well for you and you are worried about experiencing depression or anxiety symptoms again. For this reason, the best time to make shifts in the type of medication or its dosage is *before* you are pregnant. If you have the opportunity, plan to adjust your medication (come off or switch to one you can take during pregnancy) three to six months before you become pregnant.

If you've been taking antidepressants for a long time, pregnancy is an opportunity to re-evaluate your symptom management plan. The bottom-up strategies—both those you practice on your own and those you see a professional for—in the previous chapter are very efficacious, and many people find relief within a few sessions. In perinatal research, counselling therapies have been shown to be equally as effective for symptom relief as antidepressants, especially for women with mild to moderate level symptoms, and these therapies can help you sculpt new habits, thinking patterns, and relationships that are often the root cause of depression and anxiety. If you choose to stay on an antidepressant, consider combining it minimally with bottom-up brain-based strategies or therapy for faster, more complete symptom relief than medication alone might offer.

More and more, we're seeing a move toward helping people on long-term antidepressants come off their medication, with studies showing that 30 percent to 50 percent can taper off their medication gradually *without negative effects*. But before you make changes to your medication, discuss a plan to wean yourself off with your doctor. Antidepressants aren't like pain relievers such as Tylenol that work fast and leave your system fast. They take weeks to build up in your system (at which point you feel better), and weeks to leave, which is the reason for discontinuing gradually. If you stop an antidepressant suddenly, you may experience uncomfortable withdrawal symptoms (e.g., nausea, lethargy, irritability, insomnia, dizziness) or a relapse of depression or anxiety symptoms.[6] About 20 percent of individuals who take an antidepressant for 6 weeks or longer will experience some physical effects of reducing the medication. Your doctor can help you to taper off your medication gradually over a number of weeks. Because your nervous system is used to medication-assisted neuro-regulation, my suggestion is that as you taper off your dosage you also increase your usage of bottom-up, brain-based tools (e.g., the BEE Protocol) to help your system to remain neuro-regulated.

Deciding whether to stay on or go off your antidepressant before you get pregnant is one of the toughest choices you'll face. Part of a decision about medication use in pregnancy is coming to terms with what being a good mother versus being seen as a good mother is. When women worry about what others think about their decisions and what that says, by proxy, about them as a mother, it keeps them from getting help. Many women feel that being a good mother (and what is societally acceptable) is putting their child's needs first at the expense of their own. But I'm here to tell you that it is possible—and necessary—to consider both. If you are unwell, you cannot be the best version of you for your child.

When children are asked what they love about their moms, they often respond with the simplest of things, like "She loves me," "We go for ice cream together," and "We snuggle." Ask yourself: What do you need to be there for your kids? If that's getting help in ways that others might not agree with, then is their opinion valid? It can be difficult when your significant others don't support your decision to go on, stay on, or stop taking antidepressants. Your doctor and other key supports can provide information and be a listening ear, but the decision is ultimately yours.

It's helpful to think long-term about how to manage your depression and/or anxiety. Studies show that 2 of 3 women who had depression in a previous pregnancy will also experience depression in their subsequent pregnancies. As I mentioned in an earlier chapter, this reflects long-standing neuro-dysregulation. Practically speaking, you'll need to have a management plan that helps your brain and nervous system become, and stay, regulated so that your symptoms remain controlled. Stress, fatigue, parenting challenges, health issues, and relationship problems are just a few of the normal life situations we face that can trigger a relapse. So, be as intentional about managing your mental health as you would your blood sugar if you had diabetes. With a good management plan that involves bottom-up, brain-based tools and healthy lifestyle changes as a minimum, with counselling and/or antidepressants as warranted (e.g., for moderate to severe symptoms) you can reduce your risk of relapse of depression or anxiety by 70 percent. Whatever you decide, remember to put your mental health first. *Doing nothing is no longer an option. Your brain and nervous system will be impacted by your life circumstances—so take charge of what that looks like.*

What to Know About Taking Medication *During* Pregnancy

The decision about whether to take antidepressants during pregnancy is often fraught with confusion, stress, and uncertainty—mainly because myths about antidepressants cloud the decision-making process. If this is you, you've likely been told that you need to balance the risks and benefits, and for you it feels like a trade-off between your health and that of your baby with one of you "winning" and one of you "losing." I invite you to consider a win-win option where both you and your baby benefit.

Rates of antidepressant use in pregnancy are difficult to estimate, but it ranges from 2 percent to 8 percent, which is roughly the range for the incidence of severe prenatal depression and anxiety.[7, 8, 9] Many women who don't want to take antidepressants for prenatal anxiety or depression opt to simply live with their symptoms, believing that not exposing their child to medication is the safest option. But *untreated* depression carries unintended consequences.[10] In fact, our own research showed that it was women who had moderate to severe prenatal depression and who did *not* take antidepressants who had a higher risk of having a preterm or small-for-gestational-age baby—not women who had the same level of depression and *did* take antidepressants. It has raised the question in the clinical and scientific worlds: Is it untreated depression or the medication that carries the most risk?

Women who aren't engaged in any form of treatment for depression—self-managed or professional therapy, lifestyle strategies, or medication—have an increased risk of experiencing preterm delivery, low birth weight, high blood pressure, and postpartum hemorrhage, and their children are more at risk for developmental and emotional problems.[11] In a recent review of twenty-three studies, the risk of preterm birth was increased for women with untreated depression *and* antidepressant-treated depression. This increase in risk was small, and virtually the same size for both groups, suggesting that the preterm birth was more related to the depression than the antidepressants. And this is concerning because a preterm baby has higher risks of life-threatening medical problems (such as infections and lung, heart, and gut illnesses), plummeting the family into high stress, uncertainty, and fear surrounding their baby's future. Similarly, the proportion of children who experienced depression as adolescents was roughly equal for those born to mothers who were depressed and on antidepressants and those who were depressed but untreated. These findings tell us that depression symptoms carry significant long-term consequences for children.

So, doing nothing about your depression and/or anxiety is not the safest option—in fact, it's the option that carries the most risk. Brain-based and talking therapies and lifestyle changes have the least risk, and medication comes with some small risks, but none so serious that medication is not considered a beneficial treatment option—especially for women who were on antidepressants before pregnancy for moderate to severe depression or anxiety, or who have experienced one or more relapses of symptoms in the past. For these women, going off the medication may present greater risks than staying on it, so many experts recommend that they continue on them throughout the pregnancy and after the baby is born to avoid the risk of a relapse.[12] If you have had anxiety or depression in the mild to moderate range, it may be safe to come off of your antidepressant in favor of managing your symptoms through therapy and lifestyle changes.

For women who *haven't* taken antidepressants in the past but are experiencing their *first* episode of depression or anxiety during pregnancy *and* have severe symptoms, evidence-based clinical guidelines recommend that they begin antidepressants.[13]

Starting medication for the first time during pregnancy can be overwhelming. Let me assure you that you cannot become addicted to or dependent on antidepressants. Many people think that because they experience symptoms when they discontinue antidepressants, it means they were addicted, but if you had diabetes and you stopped taking your insulin, you would also experience physiological symptoms. Know that your family doctor will manage your treatment plan, and often finding the right dosage is a bit of a trial and error, so expect to have a few adjustments to your medication. And I don't want to be dismissive of the process of getting the right antidepressant in the right dosage for you. It can be a long, frustrating process of starting, adjusting, weaning, and starting again, especially because all the while you may not be getting relief.

As I said, antidepressants are considered safe for treating depression and anxiety during pregnancy. Australia's most recent Perinatal Mental Health Practice Guideline notes, "The causal link between exposure [to antidepressants] and adverse events is unclear and may be attributable to confounds."[14] In other words, in research on the harmful effects of antidepressants on the infant, it is very difficult to tease out the effect of the antidepressant on the baby from the effect of the depression. And so, it is only prudent to acknowledge that antidepressants do carry some small risks, which I'll talk about here so you can make an informed decision about your health and your baby's health.

I already mentioned the minor risk of heart malformations with paroxetine (Paxil). The most common side effect of taking prenatal antidepressants is the infant's poor transition from in-utero to life outside the womb. We know that 1 in 3 babies take a little extra time for their breathing, heart rate, and blood sugar to normalize and may need to be monitored in a special infant care unit for a few days with no lasting effects.[15] Other treatable risks include respiratory distress right after birth, which may require oxygen administration for a few minutes or hours; being born a few days early; and low birth weight deliveries of 70 grams to 200 grams lighter than average, which is about the weight of 1/3 of a cup of sugar. Neither the early birth nor low birth weight require special care in and of themselves.

There are also small risks of anxiety, depression, and neurodevelopmental problems such as autism or attention deficit/hyperactivity disorder, which as I mentioned, may be more related to the symptoms than the antidepressant.[16] I know these possibilities sound frighting—and they are—but the risk is small. For example, the proportion of children with autism and mothers who were on an antidepressant during pregnancy is 0.02 percent to 0.03 percent compared with 0.02 percent of those of pregnant women without depression *or* antidepressants.

Another risk is developmental delay, where children don't quite meet their developmental milestones on target. Again, the risk is small. A recent study from the Netherlands found that toddlers of mothers who had taken an antidepressant during pregnancy were delayed in achieving their developmental milestones by three months compared to women who had not taken an antidepressant. A study of over 13,000 Canadian mothers and their kindergarten children showed that 21 percent of children of mothers who had taken an antidepressant during pregnancy experienced developmental delay compared with 16 percent of children of mothers who had not taken an antidepressant.

Finally, there are online assessment tools and apps that can guide you through a decision-making process so that you can arrive at the best decision for you, your family, and your baby. They generally walk you through important considerations, such as the health of the pregnancy, your confidence in controlling your symptoms, and the symptom versus medication risk to your baby. These tools can be useful as a starting point as it will give you some indication of where you stand.

What to Know About Taking Medication *After* Pregnancy

I'll never forget one woman, let's call her Evie, whom I counselled through her pregnancy and after she had her baby. She had struggled with depression from the time she was a teenager and had decided she would go off her antidepressant during pregnancy. But as she got closer to delivery, she started to worry about being able to manage her new responsibilities; after all, she had struggled to keep her symptoms manageable when she was in university and under high stress with little sleep—and she foresaw the same situation as a new mother.

One of the things we talked about was how untreated depression, anxiety, and stress in the postpartum period carries risks, particularly in building the bonding relationship with the new baby.[17] Years of research have shown that untreated depression and anxiety make it difficult for women to respond sensitively to their infant's needs, and the mother and infant bonding experience can be out of sync so that the mother doesn't recognize or meet the baby's needs. This was why it was important for Evie to not simply stop taking antidepressants, but instead to replace medication with a non-medication intervention.

The considerations for taking antidepressants during pregnancy versus after pregnancy are largely the same, with the exception of breastfeeding. Many new mothers wonder whether antidepressants will affect their milk supply and worry about the effects of the medication on their baby. While a small amount of antidepressant medication does pass through the breastmilk (less than 10 percent), this is less than what your baby is exposed to in utero. Indeed, the level of drug infants receive through breastfeeding is so small that it is undetectable in their blood, which is why breastfeeding for at least six months is still the recommended form of feeding for women taking antidepressants in the postpartum period.

Postpartum Depression and Anxiety

Most new mothers with postpartum depression and/or anxiety experience the onset of symptoms three months after their delivery, and with treatment, many experience resolution of their symptoms within a few months. Indeed, the Australian guideline on perinatal mental health notes that the available evidence for SSRI use in new mothers for depression and anxiety "may improve response and remission rate at six to eight weeks."

How Long to Stay on Medication

Among new mothers with mental health problems at three months, most (60 percent to 70 percent) experience combined anxiety and depression, 23 percent to 25 percent have anxiety alone, and

13 percent have depression alone.[18] This is an important factor in deciding about treatment, because *most* women have both anxiety and depression symptoms, and recovering from combined anxiety and depression is harder and takes longer than either anxiety or depression alone. Most of the time, women are advised to stay on antidepressants for at least six months to avoid relapse.

Studies show that, in general, 1 in 3 new mothers is still in active treatment one year after they started treatment. As you know from the chapter on enduring and "under the radar" symptoms, up to 35 percent of women who have depression or anxiety symptoms during pregnancy or the postpartum period continue to have episodes into their child's adolescent years. Together, these facts suggest that women who take antidepressants beyond the postnatal period tend to be susceptible to long-standing depression either because their symptoms are moderate to severe or they are combined with anxiety.

The decision about when to stop medication can be taken in steps. You and your doctor will work out a plan to reduce your dosage, and if at any point the reduced dosage isn't giving you relief, you can always increase it again. In other words, you can start the process of weaning off your medication and reverse the process at any time.

Using medications to reduce symptoms of depression and/or anxiety is only one option of many. While many women mistakenly believe that medication is the only choice, this book is about giving you the wealth of options that lie before you as you take charge of your own mental health.

Moving Forward

Having a baby is an experience that divides our life: there is the before you had your baby, and there is after. And the in-between, the pregnancy, is the most massive transition in a family's life. And while transition comes with the challenge of newness, it is also bathed in a sense of anticipation about what the future holds and an opportunity to pivot to new things, especially those we've placed on hold. And so, when I think of pregnancy, I see it as a time of reclamation and new starts as we invest in our own and our baby's brain health. Optimizing your brain health and that of your baby is, in my view, the backbone of this book.

Talking about one's mental health is still personal and intimate, despite noble efforts of organizations to normalize mental health. This is especially true of pregnancy, where we can say that the *symptoms* of depression, anxiety, and stress are similar as in other times of women's lives but where the *experience* is vastly different. Every sign of depression or anxiety is accompanied by the disappointment in who we are as mothers-to-be, the fear of what it means for our baby's health and future, and the loss of hope in what we thought would be. This book is about breaking off the stigma that says there is something different and broken about women who suffer with mental health problems, that it means something different than having diabetes or high blood pressure. We dispel these myths with facts about how mental health problems in pregnancy are more prevalent than any other physical problem, how they most often arise as the consequences of lifelong struggles and trauma that we had no control over and that affected our neurobiology, and how they build resilience and strength—not weakness.

Remember, more women experience mental health challenges during pregnancy than we think. If you are suffering, don't blame yourself. While there are biological causes, it's life's stressors and triggers—external forces outside your control—that put you at risk. What you can control is your emotional health now: prioritize it when things are good and when they're bad. Don't write off symptoms; they are like red flags that signal something is not quite right. Know that these symptoms and their consequences are reversible and there are a number of strategies you can implement to find relief right now. There is help for you: turn to your partner and your social supports, consider therapy if you need more professional support. Medication is available and safe, often as a last resort. But it is there for you, so talk to your doctor.

This book provides all that you need to reclaim your mental health. The assessment tools are meant to shatter the confusion that most women experience when faced with feelings of sadness and worry and give you a starting point for decisions and actions. Use them as your own personal check-in as often as you like. And you don't have to fear the results because you also have a tool kit full of effective brain health strategies that span non-medication and medication, and personal and professional options. In fact, my recommendation is that you use these tools (e.g., the BEE Protocol, social support) regularly to keep your brain and nervous system tuned up. Then when hard times hit, you've already trained your brain on how to respond and you'll have greater resilience to walk through them. If you think you need extra support, don't hesitate to reach out for professional help. Your prenatal doctor or midwife is a good starting point for a discussion about what you are experiencing and what could help. You are armed now for that discussion, knowing that there are several professional options that include bottom-up (such as neurofeedback) and top-down approaches (for example, talking therapy), and medication.

One focus here has been to lay a foundation based on the neurobiology of perinatal mental health so that we can reclaim the conversation of what it means to have prenatal depression, anxiety, and stress from one of stigma and shame to the empowerment and hope that neuroplasticity offers us.

Globally, we are observing the highest rates of prenatal mental health problems we've ever seen. With all that traditional mental health care has to offer, it isn't enough to reduce or even keep at bay the number of women who suffer with mental health problems. We have untapped resources in the decades of solid research that link family-of-origin experiences, difficult relationships, attachment challenges, and toxic stress to chronic prenatal mental health problems and poor child outcomes. The question is: What are we prepared to do with this evidence? It's time to clinically acknowledge and build on the vast evidence across multiple disciplines to reposition mental health care on a foundation of neuroscience that allows us to optimize the brain health of mothers and babies.

The information, tools, and resources that this book offers are intended to help you to maintain your brain and nervous system in a regulated state, thereby reducing symptoms of depression, anxiety, and stress. The body of evidence that links dysregulation of the mother's stress system to dysregulation of the child's suggests that targeting prenatal neuro-regulation is the most direct approach to brain health for both. While I recommend brain-based tools and therapies as your core strategy, I also share how talk therapies and lifestyle changes (such as accessing social support, having better sleep, and improving your relationship with your partner) can strengthen your ability to maintain neuro-regulation at the top level of the Autonomic Ladder, lessening the risk of your biological vulnerabilities becoming realities.

While I see great potential in brain-based therapies because they offer fast, effective, and lasting results, I also see great hope for future generations. The promise of neuroplasticity is that our ACEs don't have to continue impacting us neurobiologically, emotionally, physically, and socially—and they don't have to be transmitted intergenerationally.[1] The changes early ACEs made to our genetic profile can be reversed so that our children are not at the mercy of our past experiences.

What also gives me hope is how far we've come since I began working with new mothers and families in the neonatal intensive care unit. As I have researched prenatal mental health and counselled women over the last thirty years, I've seen women that I've worked with go from suffering to thriving with the knowledge and strategies that I've shared in this book. My goal has always been to empower pregnant women to take charge of their own and their baby's mental health. And it's my hope that this book extends far beyond the small circle of women that I can reach to help many more women, babies, and families.

Acknowledgements

I have dedicated this book to my family. My husband of thirty-eight years, Robert, has been my lifelong love. We are partners in the truest sense, together bearing all the joy and losses that life has given us. Joshua and Joel, now young men, came to us after several years of infertility when we thought we would never have children. They have made our family journey rich and full. And our family's sense of togetherness has soared to new heights as we muck about on the sheep farm our family now owns and works.

My mom inspired my love of books at an early age. With the few resources she had, she made sure that I was a member of the book-of-the-month club, and I fondly remember our Saturday trips to the local library. My mom (and my grandmother!) carried a dream to write—a dream that was not realized in their lifetimes, but which has become a legacy through our son, Joshua Kingston, who is a published author, and now me with the release of this book. As I sat by my mom's bedside in the hospital the week before she died, she'd ask me for updates on the book contract. I was able to sign the contract just before she died. She was so proud that this book would become a reality. I'm truly blessed to be the daughter of parents who spoke the value of living at the outermost edges of my gifts and talents—a torch that my dad continues to carry to this day.

Not a day goes by that I am not thankful for the HOPE research team—passionate and dedicated in their support of women and their families. We have journeyed together since my early days as a junior academic. Few academics have experienced the blessing of such a magnificent team: supportive, innovative, unafraid to question, hardworking, and passionate about the women we serve. I cherish Marie, friend and confidante, whom we would all agree is the heart and soul of the team. Nikki's extreme kindness and deep love spreads across the team and to the women involved in our research. Grace's artistry and expressiveness help us to communicate ideas to women. Lindsay, now caring for her own small children, has a heart for young families that has infused our team and work with bravado and innovative ideas to push the boundaries of what families need and deserve. Dr. Kashif Mughal's statistical and manuscript work and mentorship of young researchers are key for spreading our research and inspiring clinical change. Dr. Afirah Naz, deeply committed to immigrant women's mental health, builds community and resources in places we could not reach. And above all, the HOPE team has supported each other in the journey of taking women's mental health to new levels.

The Lois Hole Hospital for Women, one of Canada's three women's hospitals, has supported the HOPE team's research throughout my academic career. They are a model example of a beautifully collaborative partnership between clinical care and research, and they continue to inspire us with their high standard of excellence of care for women. In particular, I thank long-term colleagues Andrew Otway, Sharlene Rutherford, and Lindsay Robertson, as well as the

Royal Alexandra Hospital Foundation team and the Alberta Women's Health Foundation for their support, unwavering faith in our work and team, and enthusiasm about *Your Brain on Pregnancy.*

I am grateful for Regina Ryan (Regina Ryan Books), my agent, who saw the potential and need for this book first. She has tirelessly supported this book so that it had a chance to breathe in the world.

I want to acknowledge my editors at Simon & Schuster, Sarah St. Pierre and Brittany Lavery. They have been marvellous in improving the book, making its message clearer and more impactful. And they have taught me much in the process.

There are many people who have inspired this work through their research, clinical work, insight, and integrity. Among those who have influenced me personally and professionally are Deb Dana, Dr. Henry Cloud, Dr. Stephen Porges, and Dr. Bessel van der Kolk, who have shifted the trajectory of mental health care and neuroscience. I have long admired the work of the late Dr. Bruce McEwen, who forever changed our understanding of the consequences of stress on the human body. And I am grateful for researchers across the globe who have spent their careers taking daring stances in the service of improving perinatal mental health care.

I am a woman of faith and end these acknowledgements by thanking God for the ability He has given me to do this work, and the humility to know that any good that comes from it belongs to Him.

Notes

INTRODUCTION: FIRST STEPS

1. D. Kingston, W. Sword, P. Krueger, S. Hanna, and M. Markle-Reid, "Life Course Pathways to Prenatal Maternal Stress," *Journal of Obstetrical, Gynecological, and Neonatal Nursing* 41(5) (2012): 609–26.
2. D. E. Kingston, A. Biringer, A. Toosi, M. I. Heaman, G. C. Lasiuk, S. W. McDonald, J. Kingston, W. Sword, K. Jarema, and M. P. Austin, "Disclosure During Prenatal Mental Health Screening," *Journal of Affective Disorders* 186 (2015): 90–94.
3. N. Fairbrother, P. Janssen, M. M., Antony, E. Tucker, and A. H. Young, "Perinatal Anxiety Disorder Prevalence and Incidence," *Journal of Affective Disorders* 200 (2016): 148–55.
4. D. Kingston, M. P. Austin, M. Heaman, S. McDonald, G. Lasiuk, W. Sword, R. Giallo, K. Hegadoren, L. Vermeyden, S. V. van Zanten, J. Kingston, K. Jarema, and A. Biringer, "Barriers and Facilitators of Mental Health Screening in Pregnancy," *Journal of Affective Disorders* 186 (2015): 350–57.
5. R. Webb, N. Uddin, G. Constantinou, E. Ford, A. Easter, J. Shakespeare, A. Hann, N. Roberts, F. Alderdice, A. Sinesi, R. Coates, S. Hogg, S. Ayers, MATRIx Study Team, "Meta-Review of the Barriers and Facilitators to Women Accessing Perinatal Mental Healthcare," *BMJ Open* 13(7) (July 20, 2023): e066703, doi:10.1136/bmjopen-2022-066703.

6. R. Webb et al., "Meta-Review of the Barriers and Facilitators to Women Accessing Perinatal Mental Healthcare," e066703.

7. D. Kingston et al., "Barriers and Facilitators of Mental Health Screening in Pregnancy," *Journal of Affective Disorders* 186 (2015): 350–57.

8. Z. Abrahams et al., "Facilitators and Barriers to Detection and Treatment of Depression, Anxiety and Experiences of Domestic Violence in Pregnant Women," *Scientific Reports* 13(1) (2023): 12457.

9. Y. Hu et al., "Barriers and Facilitators of Psychological Help-Seeking Behaviors for Perinatal Women with Depressive Symptoms: A Qualitative Systematic Review Based on the Consolidated Framework for Implementation Research," *Midwifery* 122 (2023): 103686.

10. R. Webb et al., "Meta-Review of the Barriers and Facilitators to Women Accessing Perinatal Mental Healthcare," *BMJ Open* 13(7) (2023): e066703.

11. D. D. Kingston, "The HOPE Platform—Mental Health for Women" (2023); available from: https://www.hopementalhealth4women.com/.

CHAPTER 1: THE RESEARCH

1. K. McKee et al., "Perinatal Mood and Anxiety Disorders, Serious Mental Illness, and Delivery-Related Health Outcomes, United States, 2006–2015," *BMC Women's Health* 20(1) (2020): 150.

2. T. A. Manuck et al., "The Phenotype of Spontaneous Preterm Birth: Application of a Clinical Phenotyping Tool," *American Journal of Obstetrics & Gynecology* 212(4) (2015): 487 e1–487 e11.

3. B. Larsen and B. Luna, "Adolescence as a Neurobiological Critical Period for the Development of Higher-Order Cognition," *Neuroscience & Biobehavioral Reviews* 94 (2018): 179–95.

4. D. Dana, "A Beginner's Guide to the Polyvagal Theory," (2022): 6.

5. J. Fisher, *Transforming the Living Legacy of Trauma: A Workbook for Survivors and Therapists* (Eau Claire, WI: PESI Publishing and Media, 2021).

6. A. Agorastos and G. P. Chrousos, "The Neuroendocrinology of Stress: The Stress-Related Continuum of Chronic Disease Development," *Molecular Psychiatry* 27(1) (2022): 502–13.

7. B. S. McEwen, "Brain on Stress: How the Social Environment Gets Under the Skin," *Proceedings of the National Academy of Sciences of the United States of America*, 109 Suppl 2 (2012): 17180–85.

8. B. A. Van der Kolk, "Developmental Trauma Disorder: Toward a Rational Diagnosis for Children with Complex Trauma Histories," *Psychiatric Annals* 35 (2005): 401–08.

9. J. Fisher, *Transforming the Living Legacy of Trauma*.

10. M. Soliva-Estruch, K. L. Tamashiro, and N. P. Daskalakis, "Genetics and Epigenetics of Stress: New Avenues for an Old Concept," *Neurobiology of Stress* 23 (2023): 100525.

11. R. C. Kessler et al., "Childhood Adversities and Adult Psychopathology in the WHO World Mental Health Surveys," *British Journal of Psychiatry* 197(5) (2010): 378–85.

12. Y. Wu et al., "Association of Prenatal Maternal Psychological Distress with Fetal Brain Growth, Metabolism, and Cortical Maturation," *JAMA Network Open* 3(1) (2020): e1919940.

13. P. R. Kaliush et al., "Examining Implications of the Developmental Timing of Maternal Trauma for Prenatal and Newborn Outcomes," *Infant Behavior and Development* 72 (2023): 101861.

14. N. Doidge, *The Brain That Changes Itself: Stories of Personal Triumph from the Frontiers of Brain Science* (London, UK: Penguin Life, 2007), 448.

15. D. Siegel, *The Developing Mind,* 3rd ed. (New York: Guilford Press, 2020), 624.

16. V. J. Felitti et al., "Relationship of Childhood Abuse and Household Dysfunction to Many of the Leading Causes of Death in Adults. The Adverse Childhood Experiences (ACE) Study," *American Journal of Preventive Medicine* 14(4) (1998): 245–58.

17. M. T. Merrick, D. C. Ford, K. A. Ports, and A. S. Guinn, "Prevalence of Adverse Childhood Experiences from the 2011–2014 Behavioral Risk Factor Surveillance System in 23 States," *JAMA Pediatrics* 172(11) (2018): 1038–44.

18. A. Wajid et al., "Adversity in Childhood and Depression in Pregnancy," *Archives of Women's Mental Health* 23(2) (2020): 169–80.

19. T. Feiler, S. Vanacore, and C. Dolbier, "Relationships Among Adverse

and Benevolent Childhood Experiences, Emotion Dysregulation, and Psychopathology Symptoms," *Adversity and Resilience Science* (2023): 1–17.

20. S. Finlay et al., "Adverse Childhood Experiences and Allostatic Load: A Systematic Review," *Neuroscience & Biobehavioral Reviews* 136 (2022): 104605.

21. N. Vyas et al., "Systematic Review and Meta-analysis of the Effect of Adverse Childhood Experiences (ACEs) on Brain-Derived Neurotrophic Factor (BDNF) Levels," *Psychoneuroendocrinology* 151(2023): 106071.

22. K. E. Wong et al., "Examining the Relationships Between Adverse Childhood Experiences (ACEs), Cortisol, and Inflammation Among Young Adults," *Brain, Behavior, and Immunity—Health* 25 (2022): 100516.

23. Z. A. Bhutta et al., "Adverse Childhood Experiences and Lifelong Health," *Nature Medicine* 29(7) (2023): 1639–48.

24. F. R. Querdasi et al., "Multigenerational Adversity Impacts on Human Gut Microbiome Composition and Socioemotional Functioning in Early Childhood," *Proceedings of the National Academy of Sciences of the United States of America* 120(30) (2023): e2213768120.

25. F. R. Querdasi et al., "Multigenerational Adversity Impacts on Human Gut Microbiome," 1.

26. E. Goldstein and R. L. Brown, "Influence of Maternal Adverse Childhood Experiences on Birth Outcomes in American Indian and Non-Hispanic White Women," *MCN: The American Journal of Maternal/Child Nursing* 48(5) (September–October 2023): E9.

27. A. L. Nowak et al., "Stress During Pregnancy and Epigenetic Modifications to Offspring DNA: A Systematic Review of Associations and Implications for Preterm Birth," *Journal of Perinatal & Neonatal Nursing* 34(2) (2020): 134–45.

28. C. L. Hemady et al., "Patterns of Adverse Childhood Experiences and Associations with Prenatal Substance Use and Poor Infant Outcomes in a Multi-Country Cohort of Mothers: A Latent Class Analysis," *BMC Pregnancy and Childbirth* 22(1) (2022): 505.

29. T. R. Foti et al., "Associations Between Adverse Childhood Experiences

(ACEs) and Prenatal Mental Health and Substance Use," *International Journal of Environmental Research and Public Health* 20(13) (July 2023): 6289.

30. B. Larsen and B. Luna, "Adolescence as a Neurobiological Critical Period for the Development of Higher-Order Cognition," 179–95.

31. E. Leavy et al., "Disrespect During Childbirth and Postpartum Mental Health: A French Cohort Study," *BMC Pregnancy and Childbirth* 23(1) (2023): 241.

32. C. Fabbri, J. Mutz, C. M. Lewis, and A. Serretti, "Depressive Symptoms and Neuroticism-Related Traits Are the Main Factors Associated with Wellbeing Independent of the History of Lifetime Depression in the UK Biobank," *Psychological Medicine* 53(7) (May 2023): 3000–08.

33. G. Sydsjo, S. Agnafors, M. Bladh, and A. Josefsson, "Anxiety in Women—a Swedish National Three-Generational Cohort Study," *BMC Psychiatry* 18(1) (2018): 168.

34. D. Zuccarello et al., "Epigenetics of Pregnancy: Looking Beyond the DNA Code," *Journal of Assisted Reproduction and Genetics* 39(4) (2022): 801–16.

35. S. Jiang et al., "Epigenetic Modifications in Stress Response Genes Associated with Childhood Trauma," *Frontiers in Psychiatry* 10 (2019): 808.

36. K. N. Fitzgerald et al., "Potential Reversal of Epigenetic Age Using a Diet and Lifestyle Intervention: A Pilot Randomized Clinical Trial," *Aging* (Albany, NY) 13(7) (2021): 9419–32.

37. M. Franzago et al., "The Epigenetic Aging, Obesity, and Lifestyle," *Frontiers in Cell and Developmental Biology* 10 (2022): 985274.

38. C. Evans, J. Kreppner, and P. J. Lawrence, "The Association Between Maternal Perinatal Mental Health and Perfectionism," 1052–74.

39. K. Limburg, H. J. Watson, M. S. Hagger, and S. J. Egan, "The Relationship Between Perfectionism and Psychopathology: A Meta-Analysis," *Journal of Clinical Psychology* 73(10) (2017): 1301–26.

40. S. J. Egan et al., "A Longitudinal Investigation of Perfectionism and Repetitive Negative Thinking in Perinatal Depression," *Behaviour Research and Therapy* 97 (2017): 26–32.

41. Y. Hamlaci Baskaya and K. Ilcioglu, "Effect of Lifestyles on Fear of Pregnancy: Development and Psychometric Testing of the Fear of Pregnancy Scale," *European Journal of Obstetrics & Gynecology and Reproductive Biology* 285 (2023): 119.

42. C. Evans, J. Kreppner, and P. J. Lawrence, "The Association Between Maternal Perinatal Mental Health and Perfectionism: A Systematic Review and Meta-Analysis," *British Journal of Clinical Psychology* 61(4) (2022): 1052–74.

43. E. Bull, S. Al-Janabi, and C. B. Gittens, "Are Women with Traits of Perfectionism More Likely to Develop Perinatal Depression? A Systematic Review and Meta-Analysis," *Journal of Affective Disorders* 296 (2022): 67–78.

44. T. Padoa, D. Berle, and L. Roberts, "Comparative Social Media Use and the Mental Health of Mothers with High Levels of Perfectionism," *Journal of Social and Clinical Psychology* 37(7) (2018).

45. B. Dobos, B. F. Piko, and D. Mellor, "What Makes University Students Perfectionists? The Role of Childhood Trauma, Emotional Dysregulation, Academic Anxiety, and Social Support," *Scandinavian Journal of Psychology* 62(3) (2021): 443–47.

46. T. Curran and A. P. Hill, "Young People's Perceptions of Their Parents' Expectations and Criticism Are Increasing Over Time: Implications for Perfectionism," *Psychological Bulletin* 148(1–2) (2022): 107–28.

47. T. Curran and A. P. Hill, "Perfectionism Is Increasing Over Time: A Meta-Analysis of Birth Cohort Differences from 1989 to 2016," *Psychological Bulletin* 145(4) (2019): 410–29.

48. R. Bunevicius, L. Kusminskas, A. Bunevicius, R. J. Nadisauskiene, K. Jureniene, and V. J. Pop, "Psychosocial Risk Factors for Depression During Pregnancy," *Acta Obstetricia et Gynecologica Scandinavica* 88(5) (2009): 599–605.

49. D. Nettle, *Personality: What Makes You the Way You Are* (New York: Oxford University Press, 2007), 298.

50. K. Fields, L. Ciciolla, S. Addante, G. Erato, A. Quigley, S. N. Mullins-Sweatt, and K. M. Shreffler, "Maternal Adverse Childhood Experiences and Perceived Stress During Pregnancy: The Role of

Personality," *Journal of Child & Adolescent Trauma* 16(3) (March 20, 2023): 649–57.

51. M. S. Conrad and E. Trachtenberg, "Personality Traits, Childbirth Expectations, and Childbirth Experiences: A Prospective Study," *Journal of Reproductive and Infant Psychology* 41(4) (2023): 403–16.

52. P. Calpbinici, F. Terzioglu, and G. Koc, "The Relationship of Perceived Social Support, Personality Traits and Self-Esteem of the Pregnant Women with the Fear of Childbirth," *Health Care for Women International* (2021): 1–15.

53. O. Echabe-Ecenarro, I. Orue, and N. Cortazar, "Social Support, Temperament and Previous Prenatal Loss Interact to Predict Depression and Anxiety During Pregnancy," *Journal of Reproductive and Infant Psychology* (2023): 1–14.

54. A. Bellomo et al., "Perinatal Depression Screening and Prevention: Descriptive Findings from a Multicentric Program in the South of Italy," *Frontiers in Psychiatry* 13 (2022): 962948.

55. G. Castellini et al., "Emotional Dysregulation, Alexithymia and Neuroticism: A Systematic Review on the Genetic Basis of a Subset of Psychological Traits," *Psychiatric Genetics* 33(3) (2023): 79–101.

56. S. I. Ahmad, E. W. Shih, K. Z. LeWinn, L. Rivera, J. C. Graff, W. A. Mason, C. J. Karr, S. Sathyanarayana, F. A. Tylavsky, and N. R. Bush, "Intergenerational Transmission of Effects of Women's Stressors During Pregnancy: Child Psychopathology and the Protective Role of Parenting," *Frontiers in Psychiatry* 13 (April 25, 2022): 838535.

57. E. Antoniou, P. Stamoulou, M. D. Tzanoulinou, and E. Orovou, "Perinatal Mental Health; The Role and the Effect of the Partner: A Systematic Review," *Healthcare* (Basel) 9(11) (November 18, 2021): 1572.

58. D. Kingston, M. Heaman, D. Fell, S. Dzakpasu, and B. Chalmers, "Factors Associated with Perceived Stress and Stressful Life Events in Pregnant Women: Findings from the Canadian Maternity Experiences Survey," *Maternal and Child Health Journal* 16(1) (January 2012):158–68.

59. D. Kingston et al., "Factors Associated with Perceived Stress and Stressful Life Events in Pregnant Women," 158–68.

60. M. K. Mughal, R. Giallo, M. Arshad, P. D. Arnold, K. Bright, E. M. Charrois, B. Rai, A. Wajid, and D. Kingston, "Trajectories of Maternal Depressive Symptoms from Pregnancy to 11 Years Postpartum: Findings from Avon Longitudinal Study of Parents and Children (ALSPAC) Cohort," *Journal of Affective Disorders* 328 (May 1, 2023): 191–99.

61. F. Vanwetswinkel, R. Bruffaerts, U. Arif, and T. Hompes, "The Longitudinal Course of Depressive Symptoms During the Perinatal Period: A Systematic Review," *Journal of Affective Disorders* 315 (October 15, 2022): 213–23.

62. M. K. Mughal et al., "Trajectories of Maternal Depressive Symptoms from Pregnancy to 11 Years Postpartum," 191–99.

63. J. Webster et al., "Measuring Social Support in Pregnancy: Can It Be Simple and Meaningful?" *Birth* 27(2) (2000): 97–101.

64. N. Smyth et al., "Anxious Attachment Style Predicts an Enhanced Cortisol Response to Group Psychosocial Stress," *Stress* 18(2) (2015): 143–48.

65. N. Smyth et al., "Anxious Attachment Style," 143–48.

66. B. H. Lipton, *The Biology of Belief: Unleashing the Power of Consciousness, Matter & Miracles*, 1st ed. (Carlsbad, CA: Hay House, 2015), xxix.

67. M. Reisi, A. Kazemi, M. R. Abedi, and N. Nazarian, "Spouse's Coping Strategies Mediate the Relationship Between Women's Coping Strategies and Their Psychological Health Among Infertile Couples," *Scientific Reports* 13(1) (2023): 10675.

68. A. Oftedal et al., "Anxiety and Depression in Expectant Parents: ART Versus Spontaneous Conception," *Human Reproduction* 38(9)(2023): 1755–60.

69. D. C. G. Mendes, A. Fonseca, and M. S. Cameirao, "The Psychological Impact of Early Pregnancy Loss in Portugal: Incidence and the Effect on Psychological Morbidity," *Frontiers in Public Health*, 11 (2023): 1188060.

70. A. Mainali et al., "Anxiety and Depression in Pregnant Women Who Have Experienced a Previous Perinatal Loss: A Case-Cohort Study from Scandinavia," *BMC Pregnancy and Childbirth* 23(1) (2023): 111.

71. A. M. Kolte et al., "Depression and Emotional Stress Is Highly Prevalent Among Women with Recurrent Pregnancy Loss," *Human Reproduction* 30(4) (2015): 777–82.

72. F. Testouri, M. Hamza, A. B. Amor, M. Barhoumi, R. Fakhfakh, A. Triki, and A. Belhadj, "Anxiety and Depression Symptoms in At-Risk Pregnancy: Influence on Maternal-Fetal Attachment in Tunisia," *Maternal and Child Health Journal* (June 16, 2023), doi: 10.1007/s10995-023-03736-y, Epub ahead of print. PMID: 37326790.

73. A. Abrar et al., "Anxiety Among Women Experiencing Medically Complicated Pregnancy: A Systematic Review and Meta-Analysis," *Birth* 47(1) (2020): 13–20.

74. M. Soliva-Estruch, K. L. Tamashiro, and N. P. Daskalakis, "Genetics and Epigenetics of Stress: New Avenues for an Old Concept," *Neurobiology of Stress* 23 (February 8, 2023): 100525.

75. R. K. Fukuzawa and C. G. Park, "Role of Intrapartum Social Support in Preventing Postpartum Depression," *Journal of Perinatal Education* 32(2) (2023): 104–15.

76. L. E. Borg and J. L. Alhusen, "A Review of Factors that Serve to Protect Pregnant and Post-partum Women from Negative Outcomes Associated with Adverse Childhood Experiences," *Maternal and Child Health Journal* 27(9) (2023): 1503–17.

77. B. S. McEwen, "Allostasis and Allostatic Load: Implications for Neuropsychopharmacology," *Neuropsychopharmacology* 22(2) (2000): 108–24.

78. M. Arshad, M. K. Mughal, R. Giallo, and D. Kingston, "Predictors of Child Resilience in a Community-Based Cohort Facing Flood as Natural Disaster," *BMC Psychiatry* 20(1) (November 19, 2020): 543.

79. B. W. Smith et al., "The Brief Resilience Scale: Assessing the Ability to Bounce Back," *International Journal of Behavioral Medicine* 15(3) (2008): 194–200.

80. S. Folkman, R. S. Lazarus, R. J. Gruen, and A. DeLongis, "Appraisal, Coping, Health Status, and Psychological Symptoms," *Journal of Personality and Social Psychology* 50(3) (1986): 571–79.

81. R. S. Lazarus and S. Folkman, *Stress, Appraisal, and Coping* (New York: Springer, 1984), xiii.

82. D. Dana, *The Polyvagal Theory in Therapy: Engaging the Rhythm of Regulation*, 1st ed. (New York: W. W. Norton, 2018), xix.

83. M. Jemni et al., "Exercise Improves Depression Through Positive Modulation of Brain-Derived Neurotrophic Factor (BDNF). A Review Based on 100 Manuscripts Over 20 Years," *Frontiers in Physiology* 14 (2023): 1102526.

84. B. Bandelow and S. Michaelis, "Epidemiology of Anxiety Disorders in the 21st Century," *Dialogues in Clinical Neuroscience* 17(3) (2015): 327–35.

85. J. A. Sturgeon and A. J. Zautra, "Social Pain and Physical Pain: Shared Paths to Resilience," *Pain Management* 6(1) (2016): 63–74.

86. R. E. Hay et al., "Amygdala-Prefrontal Structural Connectivity Mediates the Relationship Between Prenatal Depression and Behavior in Preschool Boys," *Journal of Neuroscience* 40(36) (2020): 6969–77.

87. M. C. Antonelli et al., "Early Biomarkers and Intervention Programs for the Infant Exposed to Prenatal Stress," *Current Neuropharmacology* 20(1) (2022): 94–106.

88. B. H. Lipton, *The Biology of Belief: Unleashing the Power of Consciousness, Matter & Miracles*, 1st ed. (Carlsbad, CA: Hay House, 2015), xxix.

89. E. Sulyok, B. Farkas, and J. Bodis, "Pathomechanisms of Prenatally Programmed Adult Diseases," *Antioxidants* (Basel) 12(7) (2023): 1354.

90. E. P. Davis, B. L. Hankin, D. A. Swales, and M. C. Hoffman, "An Experimental Test of the Fetal Programming Hypothesis: Can We Reduce Child Ontogenetic Vulnerability to Psychopathology by Decreasing Maternal Depression?" *Developmental Psychopathology* 30(3) (2018): 787–806.

91. F. R. Querdasi, "Multigenerational Adversity Impacts on Human Gut Microbiome Composition and Socioemotional Functioning in Early Childhood," *Proceedings of the National Academy of Sciences of the United States of America* 120(30) (2023): e2213768120.

92. E. Sulyok, B. Farkas, and J. Bodis, "Pathomechanisms of Prenatally Programmed Adult Diseases," 1354.

93. C. J. Hammer et al., "Dohad: A Menagerie of Adaptations and

Perspectives: Large Animal Models of Developmental Programming: Sustenance, Stress, and Sex Matter," *Reproduction* 165(6) (2023): F1–F13.

94. P. Scorza et al., "Epigenetic Intergenerational Transmission: Mothers' Adverse Childhood Experiences and DNA Methylation," *Journal of the American Academy of Child & Adolescent Psychiatry* 59(7) (2020): P900–P901.

95. N. K. Moog et al., "Maternal Exposure to Childhood Trauma Is Associated During Pregnancy with Placental-Fetal Stress Physiology," *Biological Psychiatry* 79(10) (2016): 831–39.

96. J. J. Muller et al., "Cardiovascular Effects of Prenatal Stress—Are There Implications for Cerebrovascular, Cognitive and Mental Health Outcome?" *Neuroscience & Biobehavioral Reviews* 117 (2020): 78–97.

97. K. O'Donnell, T. G. O'Connor, and V. Glover, "Prenatal Stress and Neurodevelopment of the Child: Focus on the HPA Axis and Role of the Placenta," *Developmental Neuroscience* 31(4) (2009): 285–92.

98. V. Babineau, A. Jolicoeur-Martineau, E. Szekely, C. G. Green, R. Sassi, H. Gaudreau, R. D. Levitan, J. Lydon, M. Steiner, K. J. O'Donnell, J. L. Kennedy, J. A. Burack, and A. Wazana, "Maternal Prenatal Depression Is Associated with Dysregulation Over the First Five Years of Life Moderated by Child Polygenic Risk for Comorbid Psychiatric Problems," *Developmental Psychobiology* 65(5) (July 2023): e22395.

99. V. Babineau et al., "Maternal Prenatal Depression Is Associated with Dysregulation," e22395.

100. M. C. Antonelli et al., "Early Biomarkers and Intervention Programs for the Infant Exposed to Prenatal Stress," *Current Neuropharmacology* 20(1) (2022): 94–106.

101. B. J. S. Al-Haddad et al., "The Fetal Origins of Mental Illness," *American Journal of Obstetrics & Gynecology* 221(6) (2019): 549–62.

102. J. De Asis-Cruz, N. Andescavage, and C. Limperopoulos, "Adverse Prenatal Exposures and Fetal Brain Development: Insights from Advanced Fetal Magnetic Resonance Imaging," *Biological Psychiatry: Cognitive Neuroscience and Neuroimaging* 7(5) (2022): 480–90.

103. L. Jelicic et al., "Maternal Distress During Pregnancy and the Postpartum Period: Underlying Mechanisms and Child's Developmental

Outcomes—A Narrative Review," *International Journal of Molecular Sciences* 23(22) (2022): 13932.

104. P. R. Kaliush et al., "Examining Implications of the Developmental Timing of Maternal Trauma for Prenatal and Newborn Outcomes," *Infant Behavior and Development* 72 (2023): 101861.

105. N. MacKinnon, M. Kingsbury, L. Mahedy, J. Evans, and I. Colman, "The Association Between Prenatal Stress and Externalizing Symptoms in Childhood: Evidence from the Avon Longitudinal Study of Parents and Children," *Biological Psychiatry* 83(2) (January 15, 2018): 100–108.

106. K. S. Betts, G. M. Williams, J. M. Najman, and R. Alati, "Maternal Depressive, Anxious, and Stress Symptoms During Pregnancy Predict Internalizing Problems in Adolescence," *Depression and Anxiety* (1) (January 31, 2014): 9–18.

107. J. A. Hofheimer et al., "Assessment of Psychosocial and Neonatal Risk Factors for Trajectories of Behavioral Dysregulation Among Young Children from 18 to 72 Months of Age," *JAMA Network Open* 6(4) (2023): e2310059.

108. D. E. Choe, L. K. Deer, and P. D. Hastings, "Latent Class Analysis of Maternal Depression from Pregnancy Through Early Childhood: Differences in Children's Executive Functions," *Developmental Psychology* 59(8) (August 2023): 1452–63.

109. S. I. Ahmad, E. W. Shih, K. Z. LeWinn, L. Rivera, J. C. Graff, W. A. Mason, C. J. Karr, S. Sathyanarayana, F. A. Tylavsky, and N. R. Bush, "Intergenerational Transmission of Effects of Women's Stressors During Pregnancy: Child Psychopathology and the Protective Role of Parenting," *Frontiers in Psychiatry* 13 (April 25, 2022): 838535.

110. S. Banti, M. Mauri, A. Oppo, C. Borri, C. Rambelli, D. Ramacciotti, M. S. Montagnani, V. Camilleri, S. Cortopassi, P. Rucci, and G. B. Cassano, "From the Third Month of Pregnancy to 1 Year Postpartum. Prevalence, Incidence, Recurrence, and New Onset of Depression. Results from the Perinatal Depression-Research & Screening Unit Study," *Comprehensive Psychiatry* 52(4) (July–August 2011): 343–51.

111. M. K. Mughal et al., "Trajectories of Maternal Depressive Symptoms from Pregnancy to 11 Years Postpartum," 191–99.

112. A. M. Kingsbury et al., "Trajectories and Predictors of Women's Depression Following the Birth of an Infant to 21 Years: A Longitudinal Study," *Maternal and Child Health Journal* 19(4) (2015): 877–88.

113. M. K. Mughal et al., "Trajectories of Maternal Depressive Symptoms from Pregnancy to 11 Years Postpartum," 191–99.

114. E. M. Charrois et al., "Patterns and Predictors of Depressive and Anxiety Symptoms in Mothers Affected by Previous Prenatal Loss in the ALSPAC Birth Cohort," *Journal of Affective Disorders*, 307 (2022): 244–53.

115. A. Wajid et al., "Psychosocial Factors Associated with Trajectories of Maternal Psychological Distress Over a 10-Year Period from the First Year Postpartum: An Australian Population-Based Study," *Journal of Affective Disorders* 263 (2020): 31–38.

116. F. Vanwetswinkel, R. Bruffaerts, U. Arif, and T. Hompes, "The Longitudinal Course of Depressive Symptoms During the Perinatal Period: A Systematic Review," *Journal of Affective Disorders* 315 (2022): 213–23.

CHAPTER 2: THE FOUNDATIONS OF
GOOD MENTAL HEALTH

1. S. W. Porges, "Polyvagal Theory: A Science of Safety," *Frontiers in Integrative Neuroscience* 16 (2022): 871227.

2. D. Amen, *Change Your Brain Every Day* (Carol Stream, IL: Tyndale Refresh, 2023), 416.

3. N. Doidge, *The Brain That Changes Itself: Stories of Personal Triumph from the Frontiers of Brain Science* (London: Penguin Life, 2007), 448

4. N. Doidge, *The Brain That Changes Itself*, 448.

5. S. W. Porges, "Polyvagal Theory: A Science of Safety," 871227.

6. Ibid.

7. D. Dana, *The Polyvagal Theory in Therapy*, xix.

8. Robert M. Sapolsky, *Why Zebras Don't Get Ulcers: A Guide to Stress, Stress Related Diseases, and Coping* (New York: W. H. Freeman, 1994), 10.

9. D. Rock, *Your Brain at Work: Strategies for Overcoming Distraction,*

Regaining Focus, and Working Smarter All Day Long, revised and updated ed. (New York: HarperBusiness, 2020), xii.

10. J. P. Lima Santos et al., "Emotional Regulation and Adolescent Concussion: Overview and Role of Neuroimaging," *International Journal of Environmental Research and Public Health* 20(13) (2023): 6274.

11. N. Fairbrother et al., "Perinatal Anxiety Disorder Prevalence and Incidence," *Journal of Affective Disorders* 200 (2016): 148–55.

12. M. R. Rubinstein et al., "Current Understanding of the Roles of Gut-Brain Axis in the Cognitive Deficits Caused by Perinatal Stress Exposure," 12(13) *Cells* (2023): 1735.

13. E. M. Sajdel-Sulkowska, "The Impact of Maternal Gut Microbiota During Pregnancy on Fetal Gut-Brain Axis Development and Life-Long Health Outcomes," *Microorganisms* 11(9) (2023): 2199.

14. A. Shields and D. Cicchetti, "Reactive Aggression Among Maltreated Children: The Contributions of Attention and Emotion Dysregulation," *Journal of Clinical Child & Adolescent Psychology* 27(4) (1998): 381–95.

15. A. Shields and D. Cicchetti, "Parental Maltreatment and Emotion Dysregulation as Risk Factors for Bullying and Victimization in Middle Childhood," *Journal of Clinical Child & Adolescent Psychology* 30(3) (2001): 349–63.

16. J. T. Kraiss, P. M. Ten Klooster, J. T. Moskowitz, and E. T. Bohlmeijer, "The Relationship Between Emotion Regulation and Well-Being in Patients with Mental Disorders: A Meta-Analysis," 102 *Comprehensive Psychiatry* (2020): 152189.

17. J. Canfield and J. Switzer, *The Success Principles: How to Get from Where You Are to Where You Want to Be,* 10th anniversary ed. (New York: William Morrow, 2015), xxxv.

18. S. R. Covey, "The Seven Habits of Highly Effective People," *National Medical-Legal Journal* 2(2) (1991): 8.

19. L. Graham, *Bouncing Back: Rewiring Your Brain for Maximum Resilience and Well-Being* (Novato, CA: New World Library, 2013), xxx.

20. N. V. Alen et al., "A Systematic Review and Meta-Analysis of the Association Between Parenting and Child Autonomic Nervous System Activity," *Neuroscience & Biobehavioral Reviews* 139 (2022): 104734.

21. M. S. Tarsha and D. Narvaez, "The Evolved Nest, Oxytocin Functioning, and Prosocial Development," *Frontiers in Psychology* 14 (2023): 1113944.

22. N. Naeem et al., "The Neurobiology of Infant Attachment-Trauma and Disruption of Parent-Infant Interactions," *Frontiers in Behavioral Neuroscience* 16 (2022): 882464.

23. N. Nakama, N. Usui, M. Doi, and S. Shimada, "Early Life Stress Impairs Brain and Mental Development During Childhood Increasing the Risk of Developing Psychiatric Disorders," *Progress in Neuro-Psychopharmacology & Biological Psychiatry* 126 (2023): 110783.

24. D. W. Eilert and A. Buchheim, "Attachment-Related Differences in Emotion Regulation in Adults: A Systematic Review on Attachment Representations," *Brain Science* 13(6) (2023): 884.

25. B. A. Van der Kolk, *The Body Keeps the Score: Brain, Mind, and Body in the Healing of Trauma* (New York: Viking, 2014), xvi.

26. H. Cloud, *The Power of the Other: The Startling Effect Other People Have on You, from the Boardroom to the Bedroom and Beyond—and What to Do About It*, 1st ed. (New York: HarperBusiness, 2016).

27. H. Cloud, *The Power of the Other*, 45.

28. H. Cloud, *Boundaries: When to Say Yes, When to Say No to Take Control of Your Life* (Grand Rapids, MI: Zondervan, 1992).

29. Nedra Glover Tawwab, *The Set Boundaries Workbook: Practical Exercises for Understanding Your Needs and Setting Healthy Limits* (New York: TarcherPerigee, 2021).

30. S. W. Porges, "Polyvagal Theory: A Science of Safety," 871227, 10.

31. B. A. Van der Kolk, *The Body Keeps the Score*, 354.

32. D. Dana and S. W. Porges, *Polyvagal Exercises for Safety and Connection* (New York: W. W. Norton, 2020): xxviii.

33. D. Dana and S. W. Porges, *Polyvagal Exercises for Safety and Connection*, 30.

34. A. M. Mahalakshmi et al., "Impact of Pharmacological and Non-Pharmacological Modulators on Dendritic Spines Structure and Functions in Brain," *Cells* 10(12) (2021): 3405.

35. V. E. Frankl, *Man's Search for Meaning: An Introduction to Logotherapy*, 4th ed. (Boston, MA: Beacon Press, 1992).

36. D. Brooks, *The Second Mountain: The Quest for a Moral Life*, 1st ed. (New York: Random House, 2019), xxxiii.

37. J. L. Burnette et al., "A Systematic Review and Meta-Analysis of Growth Mindset Interventions: For Whom, How, and Why Might Such Interventions Work?," *Psychological Bulletin* 149(3–4) (2023): 174–205.

38. G. Zeng, H. Hou, and K. Peng, "Effect of Growth Mindset on School Engagement and Psychological Well-Being of Chinese Primary and Middle School Students: The Mediating Role of Resilience," *Frontiers in Psychology* 7 (2016): 1873.

39. C. S. Dweck, *Mindset: The New Psychology of Success*, updated ed. (New York: Random House, 2016), xi.

40. K. Haimovitz and C. S. Dweck, "Parents' Views of Failure Predict Children's Fixed and Growth Intelligence Mind-Sets," *Psychological Science* 27(6) (2016): 859–69.

41. D. Dana, "The Beginner's Guide to the Polyvagal Theory."

42. H. Cloud, *Safe People: How to Find Relationships That Are Good for You and Avoid Those That Aren't* (Grand Rapids, MI: Zondervan, 1995).

43. C. A. Hostutler, T. Snider, N. Wolf, and R. Grant, "ACEs Screening in Adolescent Primary Care: Psychological Flexibility as a Moderator," *Families, Systems, & Health* 41(2) (2023): 182–91.

44. L. L. Hayes, "Psychological Flexibility Is the ACE We Need: A Commentary on ACEs Screening in Adolescent Primary Care: Psychological Flexibility As a Moderator," *Families, Systems, & Health* 41(2) (2023): 274–75.

45. O. Erduran Tekin and A. Sirin, "Rumination Mediates the Relationship Between Childhood Traumas with Cognitive Defusion, Acceptance, and Emotion Regulation: A Qualitative and Quantitative Study," *Journal of Rational-Emotive & Cognitive-Behavior Therapy* 41(April 2023): 1–28.

46. A. Han and T. H. Kim, "Efficacy of Internet-Based Acceptance and Commitment Therapy for Depressive Symptoms, Anxiety, Stress, Psychological Distress, and Quality of Life: Systematic Review and Meta-analysis," *Journal of Medical Internet Research* 24(12) (2022): e39727.

47. J. L. Rolffs, R. D. Rogge, and K. G. Wilson, "Disentangling Components of Flexibility via the Hexaflex Model: Development and Validation of the Multidimensional Psychological Flexibility Inventory (MPFI)," *Assessment* 25(4) (2018): 458–82. PERMISSION FOR USE: The MPFI scales were designed to be freely available for research and clinical use. No further permission is required beyond this form and the authors will not generate study-specific permission letters.

48. O. Erduran Tekin and A. Sirin, "Rumination Mediates the Relationship Between Childhood Traumas with Cognitive Defusion, Acceptance, and Emotion Regulation," 1–28.

49. A. Aldao, S. Nolen-Hoeksema, and S. Schweizer, "Emotion-Regulation Strategies Across Psychopathology: A Meta-Analytic Review," *Clinical Psychology Review* 30(2) (2010): 217–37.

50. A. Aldao et al., "Emotion-Regulation Strategies Across Psychopathology," 217–37.

51. D. Watson, L. A. Clark, and A. Tellegen, "Development and Validation of Brief Measures of Positive and Negative Affect: The PANAS Scales," *Journal of Personality and Social Psychology* 54(6) (1988): 1063–70.

52. H. Cloud, *Necessary Endings: The Employees, Businesses, and Relationships That All of Us Have to Give Up in Order to Move Forward* (New York: HarperCollins, 2010), 238.

CHAPTER 3: THE TRUTH ABOUT DEPRESSION

1. American Psychiatric Association, DSM-5 Task Force, *Diagnostic and Statistical Manual of Mental Disorders: DSM-5*, 5th ed. (American Psychiatric Publishing, 2013), https://doi.org/10.1176/appi .books.9780890425596.

2. S. Dekel et al., "The Dynamic Course of Peripartum Depression Across Pregnancy and Childbirth," *Journal of Psychiatric Research* 113 (2019): 72–78.

3. J. S. McCall-Hosenfeld et al., "Trajectories of Depressive Symptoms Throughout the Peri- and Postpartum Period: Results from the First

Baby Study," *Journal of Women's Health* (Larchmt) 25(11) (2016): 1112–21.

4. A. Agorastos and G. P. Chrousos, "The Neuroendocrinology of Stress: The Stress-Related Continuum of Chronic Disease Development," *Molecular Psychiatry* 27(1) (2022): 502–13.

5. A. Negele, J. Kaufhold, L. Kallenbach, and M. Leuzinger-Bohleber, "Childhood Trauma and Its Relation to Chronic Depression in Adulthood," *Depression Research and Treatment* (2015): 650804.

6. C. Pittenger and R. S. Duman, "Stress, Depression, and Neuroplasticity: A Convergence of Mechanisms," *Neuropsychopharmacology* 33(1) (2008): 88–109.

7. J. E. Khoury et al., "Trajectories of Distress from Pregnancy to 15-Months Post-Partum During the COVID-19 Pandemic," *Frontiers in Psychology* 14 (2023): 1104386.

8. M. K. Mughal et al., "Trajectories of Maternal Depressive Symptoms from Pregnancy to 11 Years Postpartum," 191–99.

9. D. Kingston et al., "Pregnant Women's Perceptions of Harms and Benefits of Mental Health Screening," *PLoS One* 10(12) (2015): e0145189.

10. J. L. Cox, J. M. Holden, and R. Sagovsky, "Detection of Postnatal Depression. Development of the 10-Item Edinburgh Postnatal Depression Scale," *British Journal of Psychiatry* 150 (1987): 782–86. Reprinted with permission.

11. K. Kroenke, R. L. Spitzer, and J. B. Williams, "The PHQ-9: Validity of a Brief Depression Severity Measure," *Journal of General Internal Medicine* 16(9) (2001): 606–13. Developed by Drs. Robert L. Spitzer, Janet B. W. Williams, Kurt Kroenke, and colleagues, with an educational grant from Pfizer Inc. No permission required to reproduce, translate, display, or distribute.

CHAPTER 4: THE TRUTH ABOUT ANXIETY

1. R. G. Hunter and B. S. McEwen, "Stress and Anxiety Across the Lifespan: Structural Plasticity and Epigenetic Regulation," *Epigenomics* 5(2) (2013): 177–94.

2. D. Dana, *The Polyvagal Theory in Therapy,* xix.

3. D. Dana, "The Beginner's Guide to the Polyvagal Theory."

4. D. Dana, *The Polyvagal Flip Chart* (New York: W. W. Norton, 2020).

5. Dana, D. "The Beginner's Guide to the Polyvagal Theory."

6. Ibid.

7. Ibid.

8. Ibid.

9. B. S. McEwen et al., "Mechanisms of Stress in the Brain," *Nature Neuroscience* 18(10) (2015): 1353–63.

10. B. S. McEwen, "Protection and Damage from Acute and Chronic Stress: Allostasis and Allostatic Overload and Relevance to the Pathophysiology of Psychiatric Disorders," *Annals of the New York Academy of Sciences* 1032 (2004): 1–7.

11. B. Bandelow and S. Michaelis, "Epidemiology of Anxiety Disorders in the 21st Century," *Dialogues in Clinical Neuroscience* 17(3) (2015): 327–35.

12. S. Grigoriadis et al., "Mood and Anxiety Disorders in a Sample of Canadian Perinatal Women Referred for Psychiatric Care," *Archives of Women's Mental Health* 14(4) (2011): 325–33.

13. E. J. Fawcett et al., "The Prevalence of Anxiety Disorders During Pregnancy and the Postpartum Period: A Multivariate Bayesian Meta-Analysis," *Journal of Clinical Psychiatry* 80(4) (2019): 18r12527.

14. S. Nakic Rados, M. Tadinac, and R. Herman, "Anxiety During Pregnancy and Postpartum: Course, Predictors and Comorbidity with Postpartum Depression," *Acta Clinica Croatia* 57(1) (2018): 39–51.

15. V. Silverwood et al., "Non-Pharmacological Interventions for the Management of Perinatal Anxiety in Primary Care: A Meta-Review of Systematic Reviews," *BJGP Open* 7(3) (2023).

16. M. Altemus et al., "Phenotypic Differences Between Pregnancy-Onset and Postpartum-Onset Major Depressive Disorder," *Journal of Clinical Psychiatry* 73(12) (2012): e1485–91.

17. S. Misri and E. Swift, "Generalized Anxiety Disorder and Major Depressive Disorder in Pregnant and Postpartum Women: Maternal Quality of Life and Treatment Outcomes," *Journal of Obstetrics and Gynaecology Canada* 37(9) (2015): 798–803.

18. R. L. Spitzer, K. Kroenke, J. B. Williams, and B. Lowe, "A Brief Measure for Assessing Generalized Anxiety Disorder: The GAD-7," *Archives of Internal Medicine* 166(10) (2006): 1092–97. Developed by Drs. Robert L. Spitzer, Janet B. W. Williams, Kurt Kroenke, and colleagues, with an educational grant from Pfizer Inc. No permission required to reproduce, translate, display, or distribute.

CHAPTER 5: THE TRUTH ABOUT STRESS

1. D. Kingston, M. Heaman, D. Fell, S. Dzakpasu, and B. Chalmers, "Factors Associated with Perceived Stress and Stressful Life Events in Pregnant Women: Findings from the Canadian Maternity Experiences Survey," *Maternal and Child Health Journal* 16(1) (January 2012): 158–68.

2. S. W. Porges, "The Polyvagal Theory: New Insights into Adaptive Reactions of the Autonomic Nervous System," *Cleveland Clinic Journal of Medicine* 76 Suppl 2 (2009): S86–90.

3. B. S. McEwen, "In Pursuit of Resilience: Stress, Epigenetics, and Brain Plasticity," *Annals of the New York Academy of Sciences* 1373(1) (June 2016): 56–64.

4. B. S. McEwen, "The Brain on Stress: Toward an Integrative Approach to Brain, Body, and Behavior," *Perspectives in Psychological Science* 8(6) (November 2013): 673–75.

5. J. P. Shonkoff et al., "Leveraging the Biology of Adversity and Resilience to Transform Pediatric Practice," *Pediatrics* 147(2) (2021): e20193845.

6. J. P. Shonkoff et al., "Leveraging the Biology of Adversity," e20193845.

7. M. Rutter, "Resilience as a Dynamic Concept," *Developmental Psychopathology* 24(2) (2012): 335–44.

8. R. A. Bates et al., "Early Childhood Stress Responses to Psychosocial Stressors: The State of the Science," *Developmental Psychobiology* 64(7) (2022): e22320.

9. Robert M. Sapolsky, *Why Zebras Don't Get Ulcers*, 4.

10. F. Shamsaei et al., "The Relationship Between General Health and Coping Style with Perceived Stress in Primigravida Healthy Pregnant

Women: Using the PATH Model," *Women & Health* 59(1) (2019): 41–54.

11. B. H. Lipton, *The Biology of Belief: Unleashing the Power of Consciousness, Matter & Miracles*, 1st ed. (Carlsbad, CA: Hay House, 2015), xxix.

12. B. H. Lipton, *The Biology of Belief*, 140.

13. M. A. Miller and R. H. Rahe, "Life Changes Scaling for the 1990s," *Journal of Psychosomatic Research* 43(3) (1997): 279–92.

14. S. W. Porges, *Effective Processing and Regulation* (Littleton, CO: Unyte), 15.

15. S. Cohen, T. Kamarck, and R. Mermelstein, "A Global Measure of Perceived Stress." *Journal of Health and Social Behavior* 24(4) (1983): 385–96.

16. S. Cohen, "Perceived Stress in a Probability Sample of the United States, in the Social Psychology of Health," in *The Social Psychology of Health*, ed. S. Spacapan and S. Oskamp (Newbury Park: CA: Sage, 1988), 31–67.

17. J. P. Shonkoff et al., "Leveraging the Biology of Adversity," e20193845.

18. B. S. McEwen, "The Brain on Stress: Toward an Integrative Approach," 673–75.

19. S. Mukherjee et al., "Antenatal Stressful Life Events and Postpartum Depressive Symptoms in the United States: The Role of Women's Socioeconomic Status Indices at the State Level," *Journal of Women's Health* (Larchmt) 26(3) (2017): 276–85.

20. S. Mukherjee et al., "Stressful Life Event Experiences of Pregnant Women in the United States: A Latent Class Analysis," *Women's Health Issues* 27(1) (2017): 83–92.

21. Y. Nomura, G. Rompala, L. Pritchett, V. Aushev, J. Chen, and Y. L. Hurd, "Natural Disaster Stress During Pregnancy Is Linked to Reprogramming of the Placenta Transcriptome in Relation to Anxiety and Stress Hormones in Young Offspring," *Molecular Psychiatry* 26(11) (November 2021): 6520–30.

22. K. O'Donnell et al., "Prenatal Stress and Neurodevelopment of the Child," 285–92.

23. K. K. Schmeer et al., "Maternal Postpartum Stress and Toddler

Developmental Delays: Results from a Multisite Study of Racially Diverse Families," *Developmental Psychobiology* 62(1) (2020): 62–76.

24. J. P. Shonkoff et al., "Leveraging the Biology of Adversity," e20193845.

25. G. Maté and D. Maté, *The Myth of Normal: Trauma, Illness, & Healing in a Toxic Culture* (New York: Avery, 2022), 87.

CHAPTER 6: UNDER THE RADAR

1. T. Field, M. Diego, M. Hernandez-Reif et al., "Comorbid Depression and Anxiety Effects on Pregnancy and Neonatal Outcome," *Infant Behavior and Development* 33(1) (2010): 23–29.

2. S. L. Farr, P. M. Dietz, M. W. O'Hara, K. Burley, and J. Y. Ko, "Postpartum Anxiety and Comorbid Depression in a Population-Based Sample of Women," *Journal of Women's Health* (Larchmt) 23(2) (February 2014): 120–28.

3. W. Qi et al., "Predictive Models for Predicting the Risk of Maternal Postpartum Depression: A Systematic Review and Evaluation," *Journal of Affective Disorders* 333 (2023): 107–20.

4. A. Wajid et al., "Psychosocial Factors Associated with Trajectories of Maternal Psychological Distress Over a 10-Year Period from the First Year Postpartum," 31–38.

5. D. Kingston, H. Kehler, M. P. Austin, M. K. Mughal, A. Wajid, L. Vermeyden, K. Benzies, S. Brown, S. Stuart, and R. Giallo, "Trajectories of Maternal Depressive Symptoms During Pregnancy and the First 12 Months Postpartum and Child Externalizing and Internalizing Behavior at Three Years," *PLoS One* 13(4) (April 13, 2018): e0195365.

CHAPTER 7: BUILDING BRAIN HEALTH

1. B. A. Van der Kolk, *The Body Keeps the Score*, 1.

2. P. A. Modesti, A. Ferrari, C. Bazzini, and M. Boddi, "Time Sequence of Autonomic Changes Induced by Daily Slow-Breathing Sessions," *Clinical Autonomic Research* 25(2) (2015): 95–104.

3. V. Pruitt, "The Basic Exercise for Vagus Nerve Stimulation and Nervous System Regulation," videos/text, cited October 10, 2021;

available from https://sevenstonesmentalhealth.com/the-basic-exercise-for-vagus-nerve/.

4. S. Rosenberg, *Accessing the Healing Power of the Vagus Nerve: Self-Help Exercises for Anxiety, Depression, Trauma, and Autism* (Berkeley, CA: North Atlantic Books, 2017), xxxv.

5. N. Güdücü and N. K. Özcan, "The Effect of Emotional Freedom Techniques (EFT) on Postpartum Depression: A Randomized Controlled Trial," *Explore* (NY) 19(6) (November–December 2023): 842–50.

6. D. Church, P. Stapleton, A. Vasudevan, and T. O'Keefe, "Clinical EFT as an Evidence-Based Practice for the Treatment of Psychological and Physiological Conditions: A Systematic Review," *Frontiers in Psychology* 13 (2022): 951451.

7. J. A. Nelms and L. Castel, "A Systematic Review and Meta-Analysis of Randomized and Nonrandomized Trials of Clinical Emotional Freedom Techniques (EFT) for the Treatment of Depression," *Explore* (NY) 12(6) (2016): 416–26.

8. N. Güdücü and N. K. Özcan, "The Effect of Emotional Freedom Techniques (EFT) on Postpartum Depression," 842–50.

9. "Music and the Vagus Nerve: How Music Affects the Nervous System and Mental Health," *Music Health* blog, https://www.musichealth.ai/blog/music-and-the-vagus-nerve.

10. R. J. Ellis and J. F. Thayer, "Music and Autonomic Nervous System (Dys)function," *Music Perception* 27(4) (2010): 317–26.

11. P. A. Modesti et al., "Psychological Predictors of the Antihypertensive Effects of Music-Guided Slow Breathing," *Journal of Hypertension* 28(5) (2010): 1097–1103.

12. J. S. Jenkins, "The Mozart Effect," *Journal of the Royal Society of Medicine* 94(4) (2001): 170–72.

13. R. H. Bind et al., "Feasibility, Clinical Efficacy, and Well-Being Outcomes of an Online Singing Intervention for Postnatal Depression in the UK: SHAPER-PNDO, a Single-Arm Clinical Trial," *Pilot and Feasibility Studies* 9(1) (2023): 131.

14. A. R. Lucas, H. D. Klepin, S. W. Porges, and W. J. Rejeski, "Mindfulness-Based Movement: A Polyvagal Perspective," *Integrative Cancer Therapies* 17(1) (2018): 5–15.

15. A. R. Lucas et al., "Mindfulness-Based Movement," 5–15.

16. D. Dana, *Audio Meditations,* cited 2023; available from https://www .rhythmofregulation.com/audiomeditations.

17. B. Battulga, M. R. Benjamin, H. Chen, and E. Bat-Enkh, "The Impact of Social Support and Pregnancy on Subjective Well-Being: A Systematic Review," *Frontiers in Psychology* 12 (September 9, 2021): 710858.

18. E. Antoniou, P. Stamoulou, M. D. Tzanoulinou, and E. Orovou, "Perinatal Mental Health; the Role and the Effect of the Partner: A Systematic Review," *Healthcare* (Basel) 9(11) (November 18, 2021): 1572.

19. D. J. Siegel and C. Drulis, "An Interpersonal Neurobiology Perspective on the Mind and Mental Health: Personal, Public, and Planetary Well-Being," *Annals of General Psychiatry* 22(1) (2023): 5.

20. J. A. Dipietro, "Maternal Stress in Pregnancy: Considerations for Fetal Development." *Journal of Adolescent Health* 51(2 Suppl) (2012): S3–8.

21. J. Dowell, B. A. Elser, R. E. Schroeder, and H. E. Stevens, "Cellular Stress Mechanisms of Prenatal Maternal Stress: Heat Shock Factors and Oxidative Stress," *Neuroscience Letters* 709 (2019): 134368.

22. C. Prinds et al., "Prayer and Meditation Practices in the Early COVID-19 Pandemic: A Nationwide Survey Among Danish Pregnant Women. The COVIDPregDK Study," *Midwifery* 123 (2023): 103716.

23. J. Fallis, "How to Stimulate Your Vagus Nerve for Better Mental Health," Optimal Living, 2017, https://www.optimallivingdynam ics.com/blog/how-to-stimulate-your-vagus-nerve-for-better-men tal-health-brain-vns-ways-treatment-activate-natural-foods-depres sion-anxiety-stress-heart-rate-variability-yoga-massage-vagal-tone -dysfunction.

24. D. M. Panelli et al., "Physical Fitness in Relationship to Depression and Post-Traumatic Stress Disorder During Pregnancy Among U.S. Army Soldiers," *Journal of Women's Health* (Larchmt) 32(7) (2023): 816–22.

25. A. R. Lucas et al., "Mindfulness-Based Movement," 5–15.

26. Ibid.

27. J. Fallis, "How to Stimulate Your Vagus Nerve for Better Mental Health."

28. C. Urech et al., "Effects of Relaxation on Psychobiological Wellbeing During Pregnancy: A Randomized Controlled Trial," *Psychoneuroendocrinology* 35(9) (2010): 1348–55.

29. D. D. Kingston, The HOPE Platform-Mental Health for Women (2023); available from https://www.hopementalhealth4women.com/.

30. A. Onofri, "Editorial: Present and Future of EMDR in Clinical Psychology and Psychotherapy, Volume II," *Frontiers in Psychology* 14 (2023): 1138153.

31. S. Carletto et al., "Eye Movement Desensitization and Reprocessing for Depression: A Systematic Review and Meta-Analysis," *European Journal of Psychotraumatology* 12(1) (2021): 1894736.

32. A. Onofri, "Editorial: Present and Future of EMDR," 1138153.

33. P. Novo Navarro et al., "25 Years of Eye Movement Desensitization and Reprocessing (EMDR): The EMDR Therapy Protocol, Hypotheses of Its Mechanism of Action and a Systematic Review of Its Efficacy in the Treatment of Post-Traumatic Stress Disorder," *Revista de Psiquiatría y Salud Mental* (Engl ed.), 11(2) (2018): 101–14.

34. F. M. Corrigan, D. Grand, and R. Raju, "Brainspotting: Sustained Attention, Spinothalamic Tracts, Thalamocortical Processing, and the Healing of Adaptive Orientation Truncated by Traumatic Experience," *Medical Hypotheses* 84(4) (2015): 384–94.

35. F. D'Antoni, A. Matiz, F. Fabbro, and C. Crescentini, "Psychotherapeutic Techniques for Distressing Memories: A Comparative Study Between EMDR, Brainspotting, and Body Scan Meditation," *International Journal of Environmental Research and Public Health* 19(3) (2022): 1142.

36. B. M. Thompson and S. R. Andrews, "An Historical Commentary on the Physiological Effects of Music: Tomatis, Mozart and Neuropsychology," *Integrative Physiological & Behavioral Science* 35(3) (2000): 174–88.

37. P. Schneider et al., "Short-Term Plasticity of Neuro-Auditory

Processing Induced by Musical Active Listening Training," *Annals of the New York Academy of Sciences* 1517(1) (2022): 176–90.

38. K. N. T. Månsson, U. Lueken, and A. Frick, "Enriching CBT by Neuroscience: Novel Avenues to Achieve Personalized Treatments," *International Journal of Cognitive Therapy* 14 (2021): 182–95.

39. N. Clinkscales, L. Golds, K. Berlouis, and A. MacBeth, "The Effectiveness of Psychological Interventions for Anxiety in the Perinatal Period: A Systematic Review and Meta-Analysis," *Psychology and Psychotherapy* 96(2) (2023): 296–327.

40. C. J. Siwik et al., "Preventing Depression Relapse: A Qualitative Study on the Need for Additional Structured Support Following Mindfulness-Based Cognitive Therapy," *Global Advances in Integrative Medicine and Health* 12 (2023), 13;12:27536130221144247. doi: 10.1177/27536130221144247. PMID: 37077178; PMCID: PMC1 0108404.

41. C. Wojnarowski, N. Firth, M. Finegan, and J. Delgadillo, "Predictors of Depression Relapse and Recurrence After Cognitive Behavioural Therapy: A Systematic Review and Meta-Analysis," *Behavioural and Cognitive Psychotherapy* 47(5) (2019): 514–29.

42. R. De Raedt and E. H. Koster, "Understanding Vulnerability for Depression from a Cognitive Neuroscience Perspective: A Reappraisal of Attentional Factors and a New Conceptual Framework," *Cognitive, Affective, & Behavioral Neuroscience* 10(1) (2010): 50–70.

43. R. De Raedt, "Contributions from Neuroscience to the Practice of Cognitive Behaviour Therapy: Translational Psychological Science in Service of Good Practice," *Behaviour Research and Therapy* 125 (2020): 103545.

44. Dennis Greenberger and Christine A. Padesky. *Mind Over Mood: Change How You Feel by Changing the Way You Think* (New York: Guilford Press, 2016).

45. F. Tauqeer, A. Moen, K. Myhr, C. A. Wilson, and A. Lupattelli, "Assessing Decisional Conflict and Challenges in Decision-Making Among Perinatal Women Using or Considering Using Antidepressants During Pregnancy—A Mixed-Methods Study," *Archives of*

Women's Mental Health (July 22, 2023), doi: 10.1007/s00737-023 -01341-0, Epub ahead of print. PMID: 37480405.

CHAPTER 8: IS MEDICATION A GOOD CHOICE FOR YOU?

1. W. Zhong, H. M. Kremers, B. P. Yawn, W. V. Bobo, J. L. St. Sauver, J. O. Ebbert, L. J. Finney Rutten, D. J. Jacobson, S. M. Brue, and W. A. Rocca, "Time Trends of Antidepressant Drug Prescriptions in Men Versus Women in a Geographically Defined US Population," *Archives of Women's Mental Health* 17(6) (December 2014): 485–92.
2. T. C. Logue, T. Wen, Y. Huang, J. D. Wright, M. E. D'Alton, and A. M. Friedman, "Continuation of Psychiatric Medications During Pregnancy," *Journal of Maternal-Fetal & Neonatal Medicine* 36(1) (December 2023): 2171288, doi: 10.1080/14767058.2023.2171288, PMID: 36710395.
3. N. T. H. Trinh, T. Munk-Olsen, N. R. Wray, V. Bergink, H. M. F. Nordeng, A. Lupatteli, and X. Liu, "Timing of Antidepressant Discontinuation During Pregnancy and Postpartum Psychiatric Outcomes in Denmark, Norway," *JAMA Psychiatry* 80(5) (May 1, 2023): 441–50.
4. F. Tauqeer et al., "Assessing Decisional Conflict and Challenges," 669–83.
5. NHS, National Health Service (UK), "Pregnancy, Breastfeeding and Fertility While Taking Paroxetine," https://www.nhs.uk/medicines /paroxetine/pregnancy-breastfeeding-and-fertility-while-taking-par oxetine/#:~:text=Paroxetine%20and%20pregnancy,paroxetine% 20have%20a%20normal%20heart.
6. A. Sørensen, K. Juhl Jørgensen, and K. Munkholm, "Clinical Practice Guideline Recommendations on Tapering and Discontinuing Antidepressants for Depression: A Systematic Review," *Therapeutic Advancements in Psychopharmacology* (February 11, 2022), 12:20451253211067656.
7. Kayla N. Anderson, Jennifer N. Lind, Regina M. Simeone, William

V. Bobo, Allen A. Mitchell, Tiffany Riehle-Colarusso, Kara N. Polen, Jennita Reefhuis, "Maternal Use of Specific Antidepressant Medications During Early Pregnancy and the Risk of Selected Birth Defects," *JAMA Psychiatry* 77(12) (2020): 1246–55, doi:10.1001/jamapsychiatry.2020.2453; X. Liu, E. Agerbo, K. G. Ingstrup, K. Musliner, S. Meltzer-Brody, V. Bergink, and T. Munk-Olsen, "Maternal Use of Specific Antidepressant Medications During Early Pregnancy and the Risk of Selected Birth Defects Antidepressant Use During Pregnancy and Psychiatric Disorders in Offspring: Danish Nationwide Register Based Cohort Study," *BMJ* 358 (September 6, 2017): doi: https://doi.org/10.1136/bmj.j3668.

8. M. Dubovicky, K. Belovicova, K. Csatlosova, and E. Bogi, "Risks of Using SSRI / SNRI Antidepressants During Pregnancy and Lactation," *Interdisciplinary Toxicology* 10(1) (September 2017): 30–34, doi: 10.1515/intox-2017-0004, PMID: 30123033, PMCID: PMC6096863.

9. A. Bénard-Laribière, E. Pambrun, A. L. Sutter-Dallay, S. Gautier, C. Hurault-Delarue, C. Damase-Michel, I. Lacroix, B. Bégaud, and A. Pariente, "Patterns of Antidepressant Use During Pregnancy: A Nationwide Population-Based Cohort Study," *British Journal of Clinical Pharmacology* 84(8) (August 2018): 1764–75, doi: 10.1111/bcp.13608, Epub June 3, 2018, PMID: 29665098, PMCID: PMC6046485.

10. A. N. Goulding, T. D. Metz, J. C. Middleton, M. C. Hoffman, E. S. Miller, T. A. Moore Simas, A. Stuebe, M. Viswanathan, and B. N. Gaynes, "Pharmacologic Treatment for Perinatal Mental Health Disorders," *Obstetrics & Gynecology* 139(2) (February 1, 2022): 297–303, doi: 10.1097/AOG.0000000000004638, PMID: 34991119.

11. A. N. Goulding et al., "Pharmacologic Treatment for Perinatal Mental Health Disorders," 297–303.

12. Ibid.

13. Ibid.

14. M. Viswanathan, J. C. Middleton, A. Stuebe et al, "Introduction," in *Maternal, Fetal, and Child Outcomes of Mental Health Treatments in Women: A Systematic Review of Perinatal Pharmacologic Interventions.*

Agency for Healthcare Research and Quality (Rockville, MD, 2021), online at https://www.ncbi.nlm.nih.gov/books/NBK570096.

15. A. C. Viguera, S. A. McElheny, P. S. Caplin, L. A. Kobylski, E. T. Rossa, A. V. Young, P. Gaccione, L. Góez-Mogollón, M. P. Freeman, and L. S. Cohen, "Risk of Poor Neonatal Adaptation Syndrome Among Infants Exposed to Second-Generation Atypical Antipsychotics Compared to Antidepressants: Results from the National Pregnancy Registry for Psychiatric Medications," *Journal of Clinical Psychiatry* 84(1) (January 4, 2023): 22m14492, doi: 10.4088/JCP.22m14492, PMID: 36602927.

16. M. Bliddal, R. Wesselhoeft, K. Strandberg-Larsen, M. T. Ernst, M. M. Weissman, J. A. Gingrich, A. Talati, and A. Pottegård, "Prenatal Antidepressant Exposure and Emotional Disorders Until Age 22: A Danish Register Study," *Child and Adolescent Psychiatry and Mental Health* 17(1) (June 16, 2023): 73, doi: 10.1186/s13034-023-00624-9, PMID: 37328889, PMCID: PMC10276495.

17. E. O'Connor, M. Henninger, L. A. Perdue, E. L. Coppola, R. Thomas, and B. N. Gaynes, "Screening for Depression, Anxiety, and Suicide Risk in Adults: A Systematic Evidence Review for the U.S. Preventive Services Task Force," Agency for Healthcare Research and Quality (Rockville, MD: June 2023), Report No.: 22-05295-EF-1, online at https://www.ncbi.nlm.nih.gov/books/NBK592805/, PMID: 37406149.

18. S. Nakić Radoš, M. Tadinac, and R. Herman, "Anxiety During Pregnancy and Postpartum," 39–51.

CONCLUSION: MOVING FORWARD

1. S. I. Ahmad, E. W. Shih, K. Z. LeWinn, L. Rivera, J. C. Graff, W. A. Mason, C. J. Karr, S. Sathyanarayana, F. A. Tylavsky, and N. R. Bush, "Intergenerational Transmission of Effects of Women's Stressors During Pregnancy: Child Psychopathology and the Protective Role of Parenting," *Frontiers in Psychiatry* 13 (April 25, 2022), doi: 10.3389/fpsyt.2022.838535. PMID: 35546925; PMCID: PMC9085155.

Selected
Bibliography

Bhutta, Z.A., et al., "Adverse Childhood Experiences and Lifelong Health."
Nature Medicine 29(7) (2023): 1639–48.

Dana, D. "The Beginner's Guide to the Polyvagal Theory," 6. 2022.

Dana, D. *The Polyvagal Theory in Therapy: Engaging the Rhythm of Regulation*, 1st ed. New York: W. W. Norton, 2018.

Doidge, N. *The Brain That Changes Itself: Stories of Personal Triumph from the Frontiers of Brain Science*. London: Penguin Life, 2007.

Cloud, H. *Boundaries: When to Say Yes When to Say No to Take Control of Your Life*. Grand Rapids, Mich: Zondervan Pub. House, 1992.

Cloud, H. *Safe People: How to Find Relationships That Are Good for You and Avoid Those That Aren't*. Grand Rapids, MI: Zondervan, 1995.

Cloud, H. *The Power of the Other: The Startling Effect Other People Have on You, from the Boardroom to the Bedroom and Beyond—And What to Do About It*, 1st ed. New York: Harper Business, 2016.

Fisher, J. *Transforming the Living Legacy of Trauma: A Workbook for Survivors and Therapists*. Eau Claire, WI: PESI Publishing and Media, 2021.

Kingston, D. "The Epidemiology of Perinatal Stress: Maternal and Child Outcomes." In R. M. McEwen, B. S. "Brain on Stress: How the Social Environment Gets Under the Skin." *Proceedings of the National Academy of Sciences of the United States of America*, 109 Suppl 2 (2012): 17180–85.

McEwen, B. S. "Protection and Damage from Acute and Chronic Stress: Allostasis and Allostatic Overload and Relevance to the Pathophysiology of Psychiatric Disorders." *Annals of the New York Academy of Science* 1032 (2004): 1–7.

O'Donnell, K., T. G. O'Connor, and V. Glover. "Prenatal Stress and Neurodevelopment of the Child: Focus on the HPA Axis and Role of the Placenta." *Developmental Neuroscience* 31(4) (2009): 285–92.

Quatraro, R. M. and P. Grussu, eds. *Handbook of Perinatal Clinical Psychology: From Theory to Practice*. New York: Routledge, 2020.

Van der Kolk, B. A. *The Body Keeps the Score: Brain, Mind, and Body in the Healing of Trauma*. New York: Viking, 2014.

About the Author

Dr. Dawn Kingston is an award-winning researcher and mental health clinician who has worked in medicine for more than twenty-five years, thirteen of those as a registered nurse in a neonatal ICU. She holds a master's in nursing and a master's in counselling. She also holds a PhD in mental health from McMaster University and a postdoctoral fellowship in mental health from the University of Manitoba. She is a professor in the Faculty of Nursing at the University of Calgary, the inaugural holder of the Lois Hole Hospital for Women cross-provincial research chair in women's mental health, and the first Canadian chair in women's mental health at the Lois Hole Hospital. She has been awarded the national New Investigator Award from the Canadian Institutes of Health Research for her work in maternal mental health. Dr. Kingston and her team are the developers of the HOPE 3.0 digital mental health platform for women, the first women's-only mental health resource offering online screening and assessment tools, information, and courses related to a variety of life situations to support women. Kingston lives in Alberta with her family. Visit her website www.drdawnmentalhealth4women.com or connect with her on Facebook @DrDawnKingston.